COMMON PROBLEMS
OF THE AGED

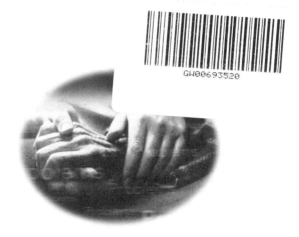

GW00693520

Edited by
Dr Chan Kin Ming

TIMES BOOKS INTERNATIONAL
Singapore • Kuala Lumpur

National Library Board (Singapore) Cataloguing in Publication Data

Common problems of the aged / edited by Chan Kin Ming. — Singapore :
Times Books International, 2001.
   p. cm.
   Includes index.
   ISBN: 981-232-133-0

1. Aged—Singapore—Social conditions.   2. Aged—Care.
3. Aged—Health and hygiene.   I. Chan, Kin Ming.

HV1451
362.6095957—dc21   SLS2001001138

© 2001 Times Media Private Ltd
Published by Times Books International
An imprint of Times Media Private Limited
Times Centre
1 New Industrial Road
Singapore 536196
Tel: (65) 2848844 Fax: (65) 2854871
Email: te@tpl.com.sg
Online bookstore: http://www.timesone.com.sg/te

Times Subang
Lot 46, Subang Hi-Tech Industrial Park
Batu Tiga, 40000 Shah Alam
Selangor Darul Ehsan, Malaysia
Tel & Fax: (603) 7363517
Email: cchong@tpg.com.my

Printed in Singapore

ISBN: 981 232 133 0

Preface

Growing old gracefully or successfully is as much an art as it is a science. Most of us dream of growing old this way, and it is not an unrealistic expectation. However, growing old is also plagued with difficulties, most of which are health-related.

Health problems in old age do not usually present themselves in a manner we expect — the so-called 'textbook' presentations. Hence, this makes geriatric medicine both exciting and challenging. When is a complaint due to sickness, and when is it due to old age? When is a complaint 'new' and when is it part of a chronic condition?

This book may not answer all the questions, but it makes interesting reading because it is based on real life patients and family situations. You may even be able to identify with some of the situations. They are all chosen to illustrate a specific problem which the lay person should know about to appreciate 'old age problems' better.

We hope that you will find this book very readable, beneficial and practical.

Dr Chan Kin Ming

This book is dedicated to all our patients,
and especially to their caregivers,
who ever so tirelessly
show love, support and compassion
for their loved ones in their old age.

Contents

1

Help! My Mum Is Losing Her Mind

Not the Same Mother

Mrs Tan, a 70-year-old widow, came to see me for 'forgetfulness' and abnormal behaviour. Her daughters, Sally and Carol, who came with her, were close to tears as they recounted how their mother was getting unmanageable, unreasonable and unappreciative of all the care she was getting. In their own words, their mother was 'not the same mother that they knew'.

I had to let them vent their frustrations before I could get them to give me a 'proper' history of their mother's problems. The sequence in which events and behavioural changes occur is crucial to making an accurate assessment and this alone will often lead to a diagnosis.

It appears that Mrs Tan was previously healthy and the happy-go-lucky sort. Widowed early at the age of 45, she worked hard as a hawker's assistant and saw her two daughters through polytechnic. She retired at 60, when her older daughter Sally got married and Carol, the younger one, started work. She was well and never needed to see a doctor. She did the cooking and marketing for the family. In her spare time, she enjoyed visiting Sally, going out with her neighbours, shopping and playing a game of mahjong every now and then.

However, about five years ago, she gradually became less interested in cooking and even stopped playing mahjong because she could not remember the cards. She also became more forgetful and would need to go to the market a few times a day because she had forgotten what she was supposed to buy. However, she could still remember the good old days and the Second World War, and kept talking about the hardships she had experienced then.

Then one day, Mrs Tan lost her way back after visiting her daughter. Fortunately for her, she had her identity card with her, and a neighbourhood police officer who found her wandering aimlessly in the street was able to take her home. Since that incident, she has not been allowed to go out of the house, and that has strained her relationship with Carol, whom she accuses of trying to harm her by locking her at home.

Mrs Tan would tell all her neighbours that she was not fed at home, although Carol was careful to ensure that she had food kept aside for her lunch. She would also pick a quarrel with Carol whenever she could not find her personal belongings and often accused her of stealing them.

Thinking that her mother was just being difficult, Carol sent her to stay with her married sister Sally for a while. This move triggered the crisis that led to her consultation. At Sally's, she walked about aimlessly, and often entered the wrong room. She started wetting herself and soiling the sofa in the house — to the annoyance of her son-in-law. It was at this point that terms like 'mad', 'senile', 'a burden' and 'troublesome' were used to describe her and the idea of sending her to a nursing home was brought up.

Doctor's Assessment

This was a previously healthy and socially active elderly person with no known past medical illnesses. The deterioration in behaviour came about gradually over a period of five years. The deterioration involved forgetfulness initially, and later disorientation to place (being lost outside the house, entering the wrong room). Then, other behavioural changes like paranoia (her daughter trying to harm her) and wandering (walking aimlessly) developed. All these symptoms suggested that she had dementia, probably from Alzheimer's Disease.

What is Alzheimer's Disease?

Alzheimer's Disease affects the functioning of the brain. Although there are no gross changes in the brain, there are abnormal microscopic depositions of plaques and tangles in the white matter of the brain. Plaques and tangles represent abnormal and degenerated brain cells (neurons).

Patients with Alzheimer's Disease are usually elderly females. Women are three times more likely to develop Alzheimer's Disease than men. Its incidence is age-associated. The mean age of onset is 78 years.

Age group	Incidence
65–74 years	about 3%
75–84 years	18.7%
85 years and above	47.2%

The disease takes a gradual and slow course initially, and usually involves loss of memory. The peculiar thing about these changes in memory is a tendency to forget recent events, while retaining a near-perfect remote memory. This is something which many caregivers fail to understand. They assume that the poor recent memory is being faked because memories of remote events are good. This adds to the misunderstanding towards persons suffering from the disease.

As the memory worsens, patients may think that others are stealing from them when they cannot find their personal belongings, or that they have been starved when they have forgotten that they had eaten. This can cause embarrassment for the family looking after them, especially when patients complain about so-called 'neglect' to their friends or neighbours.

Disorientation to place may start as getting lost after going out of the house, but may deteriorate to being lost at home. When this happens, it is usually severe. Dementia patients may not be able to find their own rooms, or the toilet (and therefore wet themselves), or they could whine about wanting to go home even though they are already at home.

Other forms of disorientation include losing sense of time or the inability to recognise a familiar person. People who suffer from disorientation to time may stay awake at night and sleep during the day, while those who are not able to recognise their loved ones may refuse to let them enter the house, thinking that they are strangers. This can be very distressing for caregivers.

The person suffering from Alzheimer's Disease has difficulty adapting to changes, be they routine or environmental. The responses to change can be confusion and agitation, wandering, or urinary and faecal incontinence. So when, with good intentions, Carol decided to send her mother to her sister's house, her mother's condition actually deteriorated. This is often seen when the elderly demented parent is shifted from one family member's house to another, which is quite a common practice in Singapore.

Although it may relieve the stress felt by each child to share the caring process, it can also put a lot of stress on the elderly parent. This is because both the daily routine and the living and room arrangements are different in each home. The same problem arises when the elderly person is discharged from hospital.

Wandering is a common behavioural symptom of dementia. It can begin when the patient is in the midst of doing something, like walking into the room to take his keys, but forgetting along the way what he was supposed to do. Wandering can also be non-purposeful walking. Wandering usually takes place when the environment is unfamiliar or no familiar persons are present.

Changes in sleep pattern may also occur in persons with Alzheimer's Disease. They may have altered sleep patterns, that is, sleeping during the day and being alert at night, shouting and being confused at night or just having difficulty sleeping (insomnia) at night. This is one of the most distressing things to happen to the caregivers as they are unable to sleep themselves, on top of having to work the next morning.

What We Can Do

It is very important for the family to understand that the abnormal behaviour of a person with Alzheimer's Disease is due to disease and not because that person is trying to make life miserable for everyone. It is not a case of 'revenge' but a genuine loss of insight by the person concerned. In the circumstances, it is true to say that the person who is suffering the most is not the patient, but the family or caregiver.

Simple loss of memory may not be dementia, but loss of memory with a change in the personality or character of the afflicted person warrants a doctor's consultation. This is because there may be other conditions that may mimic Alzheimer's Disease. Common conditions like an infection (such as influenza), side effects of drugs (like sleeping tablets or sedative drugs) or dehydration could give rise to behaviour similar to that of dementia patients.

Your doctor may need to assess whether there is any electrolyte imbalance (like too little salt in the blood), lack of certain vitamins (like B12) or a thyroid disorder that is causing the symptoms of dementia. The only way he can check this is with a blood test. He may need to do some basic X-rays or a brain scan in order to complete the assessment. In the case of Alzheimer's Disease, the results are usually all normal.

Management

Management of Alzheimer's Disease involves management of the patient and, more importantly, of the family or caregiver. At present, there are no drugs that can cure the disease. Most of the treatment is directed at managing the abnormal behaviour of the person. The various groups of drugs that have been used to alleviate the symptoms include Dihydroeorgotoxin mesylate, gingko biloba extract, estrogens, vitamins (D, E) and cholinesterase inhibitors like donepezil and rivastigmine.

Confusion, aggression and paranoid ideas are treated with antipsychotic agents like Thioridazine or Haloperidol. These drugs have side effects like dry mouth, drowsiness, constipation, stiffness and tremors, and should be used with care. For those who are often confused at night, a night light may help. Soft, familiar and soothing music in the background may be effective for agitated or aggressive patients.

When faced with an aggressive or agitated person with dementia, it is important that the family of the afflicted remains calm and reassuring. So caregivers should watch their tempers as well as loudness and tone of voice. At the same time, they need to try and find out what the frustrations are or what has brought about the emotional outburst. In some instances, distracting them may stop such outbursts from dementia patients.

For those with insomnia, sleeping tablets should be prescribed with care because some patients may react to the sleeping tablets with paradoxical agitation; in other words, they become more agitated and confused instead of being sedated. They should avoid caffeine-containing beverages near bedtime. Alcohol should be avoided too. Instead, they should do some light exercise like walking, or drink a cup of warm milk before going to sleep.

The wanderers may be allowed to wander provided they are not posing a hazard to others or to themselves. Therefore, the

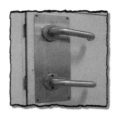

Double lock, double security

environment may have to be modified so that they can wander safely. This includes adequate lighting and non-slippery floors that are free of obstructions such as toys lying free on the floor, throw rugs, and other such objects. For those with a tendency to wander out of the house and thus risk getting lost, the door can be disguised by putting a chair or plant in front of it. Alternatively, it can be fixed with a double lock.

You may also want the person with dementia to wear an identification tag around the neck or pinned to the garment. This tag should contain the person's name, and the name and contact number of a next-of-kin. In the event that he or she is lost, at least the person can be identified, and the relatives informed.

Memory and orientation can be improved by repetition. It is important to repeatedly remind someone with Alzheimer's Disease who and where he is, what time of the day it is, and what is happening in the surroundings. This is called reality orientation. It can enhance the level of daily functioning and selfcare. Because of the limited memory, allow the person to leave things where he usually puts them.

Encourage him to remain mentally active with activities like reading a newspaper, watching television, listening to the radio, or maintaining a hobby.

Do not overload the patient's mind with information. Ask one question or make one request at a time, rather than pose a few questions together. A lot is learned by observing the behaviour of the person with Alzheimer's Disease. After a while, the family or caregiver may be able to see a pattern in the behaviour, and so be able to avoid actions or activities that are likely to agitate.

Advice for the Caregiver

Seek help early. Do not attempt to carry the burden of caregiving alone. Caring for a person with dementia is a 36-hour-a-day job. So, join a support group where you can discuss and share your problems with other caregivers. This can greatly reduce the stress you are going through, and at the same time give you some tips from those who have gone through the situations that you may be facing currently.

Allow someone to come and 'granny sit' for you so that you can have some social life. You may also consider sending your elderly relative to a day care centre or arranging for a respite care stay at a community hospital or nursing home. Going it alone can only lead to early burnout, and even to elder abuse.

Where to Seek Help

You should consult your general practitioner or polyclinic first if you notice a deterioration of memory and behaviour in your elderly loved ones. They will be able to give a general medical assessment to exclude the common illnesses that may mimic dementia. If necessary, your doctor can refer you to a geriatric specialist for a full assessment. Assessment clinics are available at these places:

Alexandra Geriatric Centre, Alexandra Hospital.

Department of Geriatric Medicine, Tan Tock Seng Hospital

Division of Geriatric Medicine, Changi General Hospital

Gleneagles Medical Centre

HMI Balestier Hospital

Day Care Centres for Patients with Dementia

New Horizon Centre (Toa Payoh)
Blk 151 #01-468, Lor 2 Toa Payoh, Singapore 310151.
Telephone: 3538734

New Horizon Centre (Bt Batok)
Blk 511 #01-211, Bt Batok St 52, Singapore 650511.
Telephone: 5659958

Apex Harmony Lodge
10 Pasir Ris Walk (off Pasir Ris Drive), Singapore 518240.
Telephone: 5852265

Thong Teck Home Day Care Centre
91 Geylang East Ave 2, Singapore 523941. Telephone: 8460069

Respite Care Services

St Andrew's Community Hospital
1 Elliot Road, Singapore 458686. Telephone: 2419956

St Luke's Hospital for the Elderly
Bukit Batok St 11, Singapore 659674. Telephone: 5632281

Ang Mo Kio Community Hospital
17 Ang Mo Kio Ave 9, Singapore 569766. Telephone: 4541729

Kwong Wai Shiu Hospital
705 Serangoon Road, Singapore 328127.
Telephone: 2993747/2945637

If you would like more information about support groups, you may contact one of the Day Care Centres for Patients with Dementia or Singapore Action Group for Elders (SAGE) Counselling Centre, Telephone: 1800 3538633, or the Tsao Foundation, Telephone: 4332740.

2

But It's Only A Fall

Falling without Good Reason

"My Mum's had a fall!" This is a very common complaint of children when they come with their aged parents to see me. Mrs Choo, who is 76, is one such person. Initially, her children were concerned. But when she kept falling and falling, and did not seem to suffer any serious bodily injuries, they became 'immune' to these falls and viewed them as part and parcel of her daily routine. Her children even hired a maid to make sure she did not need to walk and thus risk falling and hurting herself.

After a fall which happened two days before she came to see me, she complained of pain in her back and right hip. To stop her from moaning and groaning, the children came with her to see me. The problem of falling first started almost three years ago, when at age 73, she started having falls 'without a good reason'. It was attributed to carelessness, and Mrs Choo was often scolded by her children for not paying attention to what she was doing.

Doctor's Assessment

While falls are common in the elderly, the causes of falls and the injuries sustained in each elderly person are different. The doctor's approach is three-pronged:

1. Assessment of extent of injuries,

2. Determining the cause of the falls, and
3. Preventing future falls.

To assess the extent of injuries, a full examination is required to determine any external soft tissue injuries (like cuts and bruises). The presence of bruises may hide something more sinister underneath — a fractured bone, for example. So I needed to check the whole body for fractures. In Mrs Choo's case, there was pain in her back and right hip. She was lying on her left side, grimacing in pain. I gently pressed on her spine to look for localised spinal tenderness and muscle spasms along the spine. If either of these was present, it could indicate fracture of the vertebral body. Her right leg was shortened (compared to the left) and internally rotated. This resting posture of the leg indicated that she had sustained a fracture of the femur, possibly at the neck.

Mrs Choo remained very alert and rational during the examination. There were no bruises or cuts on her head, so there was nothing to suggest any head injuries that I had to be mindful of. X-rays of her hip subsequently confirmed a fracture at the neck of the right femur, and she required an operation to fix the hip. X-rays of her spine were normal.

Fixing the fracture is just one step in the management of someone who has fallen. If we do not understand why a person fell in the first place, we would not be able to prevent future falls. So back I went to investigate in detail the events related to Mrs Choo's history of falls. I was looking for a common pattern. As I spoke to Mrs Choo and her family, this pattern emerged. Most of the falls occurred when she was about to get on or off the toilet seat, on stairs and after prolonged lying in bed. Each time, she knew she was going to fall because she felt dizzy, but was not fast enough to right herself. She had also fallen in the toilet a number of times because the floor was wet, and she had not bothered to switch on the light because she thought she would not take long. On another occasion, she had fallen in the bath when she rested her weight on a towel rack, and it gave way.

Given this history, I went on to examine Mrs Choo. What struck me about Mrs Choo was that she is rather tall but thin — 1.68 m and weighing 42 kg. In a supine or lying position, her blood pressure was 130/76 mmHg, but this dropped to 80/60 mmHg when she assumed a sitting posture. This drop of blood pressure with a change of posture indicated that Mrs Choo had postural hypotension, a condition defined as a drop of more than 20 mmHg in pressure with a change in posture. It was therefore not surprising when she complained of dizziness on sitting or standing, especially after prolonged lying in bed.

In addition, I found that she was stiff in the limbs and had tremors in her hands, which suggested to me that she was suffering from mild Parkinson's Disease. Examination of her knees also showed deformed looking knees with crepitus (clicking of the knee joints during movement), which suggested osteo-arthritis of the knees. This, together with Parkinson's Disease, was probably responsible for the falls that occurred whenever she attempted to get on or off the toilet seat.

The Problem with Falls

It is easy to understand that physical injuries like fractures and bruises caused by falls are a real problem. But studies also show that the majority of falls do not result in serious physical injury. Falls incapacitate the elderly person and the family quietly with fear. This usually results in the psychological '3Fs (Fear of Further Falling) syndrome'. The elderly person may fear the next fall and its consequences and thus voluntarily restrict his/her own activities. Similarly, the family, fearing the next fall, may impose restrictions on the activities of the elderly. Either of these reactions is counterproductive. Reducing activity makes the elderly person lose confidence in his ability to walk. There is

How to Get Up from the Floor after a Fall

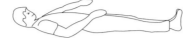

Lie on your back.

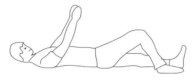

Grasp your arms. Bend one leg. Prepare to turn.

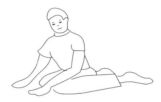

Move into a sitting position.

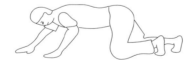

Move body forward into the four-point kneel.

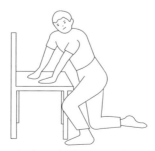

To move into the two-point kneel, place your hands on the chair. Push with hands to stand up and then turn to sit on the chair.

further loss of muscle tone and muscle strength as elderly persons begin to spend more time in bed. In fact, they lose three to five per cent muscle tone for each day of bed rest. In addition, there is loss of muscle bulk when the muscles are not exercised as well as loss of bone density with immobilisation. All these factors set off a perpetual spiral that will further increase the risk of falls and the resulting injuries.

What We Can Do

Having seen that Mrs Choo's falls were due to a combination of postural hypotension, Parkinson's Disease and osteoarthritis of the knees, I had to organise management according to priority. The first priority was to fix the fracture to reduce pain and restore function. Next, we needed to treat the underlying conditions listed above, teach safety awareness to the patient and her family and enhance safety in the home environment.

Management

For Parkinson's Disease, Mrs Choo was treated with drugs containing levodopa, like Madopar or Sinemet. This medication would reduce the stiffness in her limbs and make walking easier. To relieve postural hypotension, I advised her to increase her salt intake, and to sleep with her head elevated to about 20 to 30 degrees. Pulling a pair of tights over her legs just before she got up from bed could be effective in reducing the drop in blood pressure on sitting or standing up. If all these measures failed, a small dose of medication (like Fludrocortisone) to retain salt and induce peripheral vasoconstriction might be prescribed. Salt increases blood volume, and this, combined with the constriction of arteries in the peripheral areas of circulation such as the limbs, increases blood pressure. The usual advice — to allow the blood pressure to stabilise first before moving after a change in posture — is still relevant.

Mrs Choo was required to go for a course of rehabilitation to improve her lower limb strength and balance. To improve her confidence in walking, she was also taught how to get up after a fall. She was also assessed for suitable mobility aids such as a quad stick or a walking frame to improve balance.

Changes to the environment are equally important. The environment can make or break the elderly. Simple things that are taken for granted go a long way in making it safe for the elderly. They include:

- Adequate area lighting
- Suitable height of chairs and toilet seats
- Keeping obstacles like toys off the floor.

The heights of beds, chairs, sofas and toilet seats should be suited to the build of the person. A tall person should have a correspondingly higher chair, bed and toilet seat. If the height of a seat is too low for a person, he will have difficulty in getting up from a sitting position, and that action may predispose him to falls. Similarly, a short person should have a lower than average bed, chair and toilet seat to reduce the hazard of climbing up and down.

Mrs Choo, who is tall, has an excessively low toilet seat which caused her to fall a number of times while she was trying to get up. Grab bars or sturdy furniture, when placed strategically, can prevent falls by giving support to the elderly person at a crucial time. It is important to differentiate between grab bars which are purpose-built, from towel racks, which are secure only for towels. The elderly should never compromise by using a towel rack for a grab bar, as Mrs Choo did, with dire consequence. See the 'Checklist for an Elder-friendly Home' on page 26.

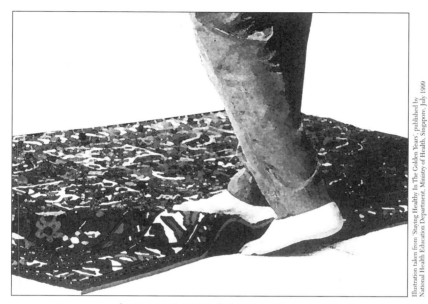

Loose rugs cause dangerous trips.

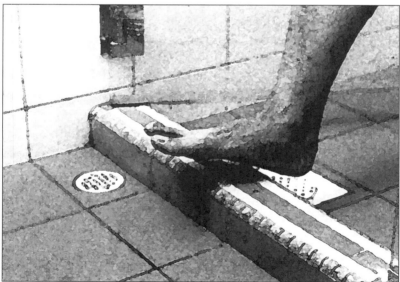

Avoid having raised dividers. Where one is present, for example, at the edge of the shower area, highlight it with bright tape to prevent tripping.

Illustration taken from 'Staying Healthy In The Golden Years', published by National Health Education Department, Ministry of Health, Singapore, July 1999

Illustration taken from 'Staying Healthy In The Golden Years', published by National Health Education Department, Ministry of Health, Singapore, July 1999

Where to Seek Help

All older persons who suffer from frequent falls should be rehabilitated, either as inpatients in a hospital such as a community hospital, or as outpatients in a day care centre. The day centres that offer rehabilitation programmes are listed on page 119.

During the period that the person is not at a day care centre, that is, at home, some emergency plans should be made in the event of a fall. This could be an informal arrangement for neighbours to check in regularly, or by some alert system. Some companies have come up with remote control pendants which elderly persons can wear around their necks or waists. After sustaining a fall, they could press on the alarm button, which connects them through a phone to their children's or designated caregiver's office, pager or handphone.

Appropriate equipment and aids should always be used to ensure safety. Instead of buying such aids or appliances off the shelf without prior knowledge of their suitability or use, get the advice of a physiotherapist or occupational therapist. Visit an independent living centre (listed below) to view the range of equipment available before investing in the equipment. The right piece of equipment, be it an aid or appliance, will go a long way to ensuring independence and safety in mobility. For Mrs Choo, it was recommended that her toilet seat be raised with a toilet seat raiser, and a set of grab bars be put up in the toilet and bath.

Independent Living Centres

Alexandra Independent Living Centre
Alexandra Hospital. Tel: 4708423

Home Care Place
Changi General Hospital. Tel: 8501868

Do's and Don'ts After a Fall

DO	DON'T
1. Reassure the fallen person.	Be too anxious and cause fear and panic.
2. Observe consciousness level, that is, whether the person is alert or drowsy.	Have people crowding around the person who has had a fall. He or she needs oxygen too!
3. Ask how the person feels, in particular: • Any chest pain or discomfort • Any difficulty in breathing • Any pain in the following areas: the head (if there is head injury), neck, back and hips. Pain at these sites may imply serious bone injuries like fractures, and the person should not be moved until professional help arrives.	Ignore complaints of the person who has fallen.
4. Allow the fallen person to move his or her own limbs and body. Inability to move certain parts of the body may imply serious injuries like fractures or nerve injuries.	Be too hasty about moving the fallen person, for example, to help him or her to sit or stand up. Any bone or nerve injuries not handled properly may worsen.
5. Ensure privacy, even if the victim is lying on the floor.	Overexpose the person.
6. If the person is drowsy, turn him or her gently to one side, and remove any dentures or food from the mouth.	If the person is drowsy, give drinks orally, unless it is safe to do so.
7. Let the victim who is immobile and in pain lie down in a comfortable position on the floor until help arrives.	Lie a person flat on the back when drowsy. There is danger of choking on saliva.
8. Call for help if you are not sure what to do.	

Affordable Homecare Aids for the Homebound

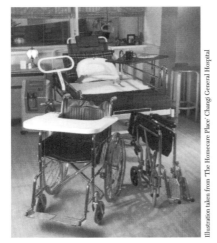

Chrome wheelchairs

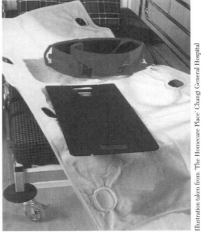

A canvas carry sheet comes in handy in an emergency.

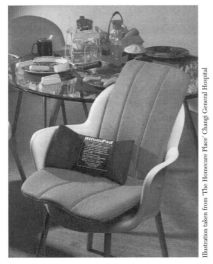

BifomPad for neck comfort

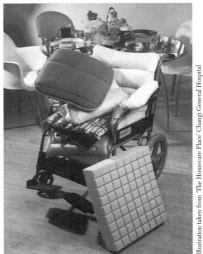

All kinds of pressure relief cushions

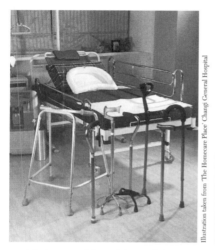

Various walking aids: walking frames, quad sticks, walking sticks.

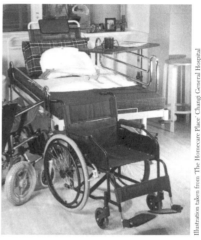

Lightweight wheelchairs (foreground)

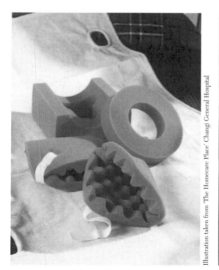

Foamy protectors and positioners offer protection from pressure sores.

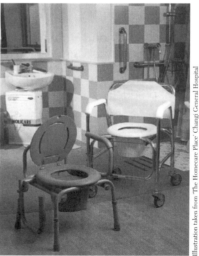

Commodes cut down on trips to the toilet.

Range of Useful Products on Display at Independent Living Centres

1. **Bed and Accessories**: beds, mattresses and other accessories

2. **Pressure Relief Products**: mattresses, cushions, joint protectors

3. **Chairs and Chair Accessories**: reclining chairs, raising blocks, footstools, backrest cushions

4. **Hoists and Lifting Equipment**: mobile, fixed and electric hoists, transferring equipment

5. **Eating and Drinking Appliances**: special cutlery, plates, cups, trays, bibs

6. **Dressing Aids**: buttoning aid, sock aid, dressing stick

7. **Toilet Aids**: commodes, bedpans, urinals, toilet rails

8. **Mobility Aids**: standing and walking frames, tripods, sticks, wheelchairs

9. **Kitchen and Household Appliances**: door openers, can openers, tap turners, key turners, electrical switches

10. **Continence Management Aids**: pads, pants and drainage products

Checklist for an Elder-friendly Home

1. **Living Room**
   a) Buy furniture with smooth rounded edges, and heavy chairs with good back support that will not topple over when you sit.
   b) Armchairs help a person get up easily.
   c) Keep rugs flat, and secure wall-to-wall carpeting firmly.
   d) Practise good housekeeping — keep floor clean and free of clutter.

2. **Bedroom**
    a) Have a light switch at the entrance so that there is never a need to walk into or through a dark room.
    b) Have a night light just next to your bed in case you have to wake up in the night.
    c) Access to the bathroom should be short, direct and clear of furniture.
    d) A bedside table is useful for holding medicines, glasses, water and other items. You should turn on the light and put on your glasses when taking medication at night. Only medication for the night should be at the bedside.
    e) Install a call-bell or have a hand-held bell in your room in case you need to call for help.

3. **Bathroom/Toilet**
    a) Install grab bars or handrails in the shower, on walls around the bathtub and alongside the toilet.
    b) Use non-skid flooring, safety strips or place a non-skid mat on the floor of your bathtub or shower.
    c) If you shower, install a non-skid shower seat and hand-held shower head so that you can sit while bathing.
    d) Keep the rest of the bathroom dry, using shower curtains or sliding screens.
    e) Highlight the threshold of the shower area to prevent tripping.
    f) Use plastic or disposable cups; glass tumblers may break when dropped.

4. **Kitchen**
    a) Highlight stove dials clearly.
    b) Store commonly used items within easy reach to avoid bending or climbing.

5. **Stairs**
    a) Install handrails and always hold on to them when using the stairs.
    b) Make sure there is a light switch at the top and bottom of each staircase, and ample lighting throughout the house.
    c) Place a strip of bright tape at the edge of hard-to-see steps and at the top and bottom step of each staircase.
    d) Ensure that stairs are free of clutter to permit unobstructed movement.

3

Spinning Out Of Control

Many Causes of Giddiness

Giddiness or dizziness is a very common complaint in older persons. It is also one of the most difficult complaints to manage. Very often, the description of what they feel is vague and confusing. It may range from a sensation of floating in the air, walking on a cloud, to just lightheadedness or an actual sensation of spinning around (also known as vertigo).

The symptoms of giddiness are very significant because they may be uncomfortable or associated with nausea and poor appetite, and therefore impair the quality of life. Giddiness also encourages dependency and a reluctance to move about. In severe cases, it may precipitate falls. Hence it is very important to know exactly what the patient means when he or she complains of giddiness.

There are many causes of giddiness. Many of my patients say that certain 'heaty' or 'cooling' foods can trigger an attack of giddiness. However, there is no definite scientific basis for this. The following patients will help to illustrate the more common causes of giddiness.

Giddiness Because Of Low Blood Pressure

Mr Lim, a 78-year-old gentleman, had been seeing me at my clinic for giddiness for the past six months. His giddiness came on insidiously and was described as a lightheaded feeling. It occurred about once or twice a week and usually came on when there was a change of posture, such as when getting up from bed in the morning, while walking to the toilet or when standing up from a sitting position. These attacks made him unsteady on his feet, but he did not fall. Mr Lim has had a history of diabetes and high blood pressure for the past 15 years, and he was on medication prescribed by his regular neighbourhood doctor.

From Mr Lim's description, it appeared that he experienced giddiness or lightheadedness whenever there was a change in posture. I felt that the most likely cause of this symptom was postural hypotension, a condition in which there is a drop in blood pressure when the person assumes an upright posture. This drop in blood pressure leads to giddiness or lightheadedness because of a decrease in blood flow to the brain. It may be precipitated when the person rises suddenly from a recumbent or sitting position.

In normal individuals, there are reflexes which prevent a drop in blood pressure when a person sits down or stands up. These reflexes are defective in persons with certain medical conditions such as diabetes mellitus, alcoholism and Parkinson's Disease. Drugs for high blood pressure or heart failure (anti-hypertensives, diuretics) are also common causes of postural hypotension. Mr Lim had had a long-standing history of diabetes and was also being treated for high blood pressure, both of which may lead to postural hypotension.

Another possible cause of giddiness is hypoglycaemia, a condition in which the blood sugar level is low. This could result when a person with diabetes has eaten insufficiently (for example, skipped a meal or has not been eating well) or has taken a higher dose of a diabetic drug. Other than giddiness, hypoglycaemia may be associated with blurring of vision, confusion, sweatiness, tremors, tachycardia (fast heartbeat), hunger pangs and anxiety.

When I examined Mr Lim, I found that he had a supine (lying down) blood pressure of 150/80 mmHg. This fell to 120/60 mmHg on standing, and he also complained of the same lightheadedness that he had earlier described. This confirmed a diagnosis of postural hypotension. His blood sugar test was also normal, excluding hypoglycaemia as a cause. When I checked his medication, I found that he was on 10 mg of nifedipine three times a day and 100 mg of atenolol once daily, for hypertension. Both drugs can cause a drop in blood pressure.

I decided to stop one of the antihypertensive tablets (nifedipine) and monitor his blood pressure closely. His symptoms improved and blood pressure was stabilised at 155/80 mmHg (when supine) and 140/80 mmHg (on standing). In addition to altering his medication, I also advised Mr Lim to adopt simple precautionary measures like taking small frequent meals (heavy meals tend to accentuate a drop in blood pressure), avoiding alcohol, and getting up from a supine or sitting position slowly (to allow for stabilisation of blood pressure).

How to Get Up from a Supine Position

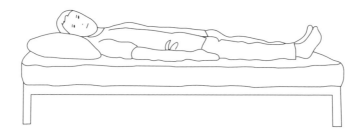

1. Turn the head towards the side on which you want to get up.

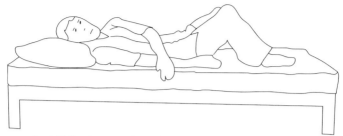

2. Lift the knees, place the feet flat on the bed. Cross one arm over the body so that it rests on the edge from which you are getting up.

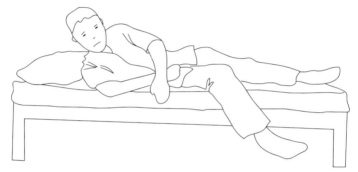

3. Lower the legs onto the floor one at a time.

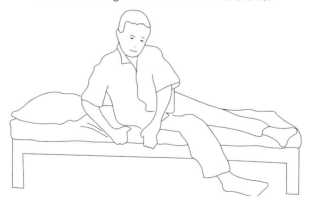

4. Meanwhile, raise the head and push up with the other hand, pressing on the elbow and forearm. The weight of the legs will help in achieving an upright sitting position.

Giddiness from Ear Disease

Sixty-nine-year-old Madam Tan was admitted to hospital with severe giddiness. Upon waking up in the morning, she felt a sudden spinning sensation as she was getting out of bed. It was a sensation she had never felt before — the whole room appeared to be swirling around in circles, and she felt as though she were about to be thrown onto the floor. This lasted about half a minute, and after that she could not walk steadily and even vomited twice when she tried taking a bowl of porridge for lunch.

Her worried son took her to a hospital as she had not eaten anything the whole day and was not better by the evening. Madam Tan did not have any known medical problems and was not on any regular medication.

When I saw Madam Tan in the ward, she was lying in bed with her eyes closed. She was very tense and afraid to move her head for fear that it might bring on an attack of giddiness. Upon close questioning, I learned that she had suffered a bout of influenza with a cough and sore throat about one week before the attack of severe giddiness.

The symptoms Madam Tan described were caused by vertigo, which is giddiness associated with a spinning sensation (vertiginous giddiness) and difficulty in maintaining balance and equilibrium. There are many causes of vertiginous giddiness. These include benign paroxysmal positional vertigo (BPPV), vestibular neuritis, Meniere's Disease and cerebellar stroke. In Madam Tan's case, her vertigo attacks were caused by vestibular neuritis, which is characterised by a sudden attack of vertigo associated with nausea and vomiting. The vertigo is not associated with hearing loss or tinnitus (ringing sound in the ear). It is worsened by nonspecific movements like sitting down or standing up, and not by specific positions of the head as seen in BPPV.

Vertigo is caused by a viral inflammation of the vestibular nerve, which is linked to balance. Madam Tan's viral attack probably came on during her recent upper respiratory tract infection (she had a cough and a sore throat). The attack is usually self-limiting and drugs are used to control the vertigo initially. Most patients recover within one week.

Benign paroxysmal positional vertigo (BPPV) is vertigo that is brought on suddenly by movements of the head, commonly when turning over in bed (with the affected ear facing downwards) or tilting the head up or down. During these movements, there is displacement of tiny crystals into the balance canals of the inner ear. These crystals settle onto specialised hair cells and stimulate the balance nerve inappropriately, leading to vertigo and unsteadiness. The attacks of vertigo usually end after six months. Treatment includes the use of drugs such as Stemetil, Sturgeon or Betahistine to suppress the vertigo, and special re-positioning exercises that move the crystals away from the inner ear canal.

Meniere's Disease is characterised by bouts of severe vertigo associated with fluctuating hearing loss and tinnitus (ringing sound in the ear). It is a degenerative disease and is most common in the fifth and sixth decades of life. The underlying cause is an increase in fluid pressure in the inner ear. Treatment of this condition is usually medical, with the use of drugs to control the vertigo as well as drugs such as vasodilators and diuretics to regulate the inner ear pressure. Occasionally, surgical treatment may be necessary. For example, a small operation is performed behind the ear to drain the fluid. Patients with Meniere's Disease should avoid caffeine and nicotine.

Occasionally, a stroke in the cerebellum (that is, blockage of blood flow or bleeding in the cerebellum) can cause vertigo, severe nausea and vomiting, headache and an unsteady gait. To diagnose this condition, you need a thorough examination of the nervous system as well as a brain scan. Treatment options include the prescription of aspirin tablets to reduce the risk of another stroke, and physiotherapy to improve balance and gait. If there is bleeding, surgery may be required.

I advised Madam Tan to rest in bed and also prescribed medication for her giddiness and vomiting. When I saw her again the next morning, she was much better and was able to sit up in bed. With encouragement, she could walk a short distance, although she was still apprehensive and unsteady. Her appetite had also improved, but there was some residual nausea. She was referred to the physiotherapist for walking exercises to help build up her confidence.

At the end of one week, she was almost back to normal and was discharged. When I saw her in the clinic one month later, Madam Tan was cheerful and well. There were no more attacks of giddiness.

Giddiness Due To 'Old Age' or Multiple Sensory Deficits

Madam Lee, who is 80, was referred to my outpatient clinic by her family doctor, to whom she had complained of occasional bouts of dizziness over the past two years. In fact, the dizziness had worsened in the past six months. Her family doctor had seen her three times, each time prescribing a different medication, but Madam Lee's condition had not improved.

During the last visit, she told him that she had felt dizzy and unsteady as she was walking to the toilet, and hence had fallen. This prompted the referral. Madam Lee had had diabetes mellitus for the past 30 years and had been taking her medication faithfully. Her blood sugar levels were well controlled. There were no other medical problems. She lived with her son and his family in a five-room flat and rarely ventured out.

When I probed further, Madam Lee could not describe the nature of her dizziness very well. She could only say that she felt dizzy and unsteady on her feet, usually when standing or walking.

There was no vertigo, nausea or vomiting, and she had never lost consciousness. After a physical examination, I found that Madam Lee had poor eyesight due to cataracts affecting both eyes. She also experienced numbness in both feet, which is a complication of long-standing diabetes.

When asked to walk, she took small steps and appeared cautious and apprehensive, constantly looking for things to hold on to. Her blood pressure did not drop after she stood up, so her dizziness was unlikely to be due to postural hypotension. I could not detect any signs that might suggest disease of the inner ear or cerebellum, both of which are important organs in the control of balance.

Giddiness is one of the most common complaints among the elderly. In some of these patients, no definite cause for the giddiness is found even after thorough physical examination and many investigations have been performed. These patients may be diagnosed to have dysequilibrium of ageing, which is the sense of imbalance due to the effects of old age.

Madam Lee's complaints of dizziness and sense of imbalance on walking are characteristic of dysequilibrium of ageing. Vertigo and hearing loss may or may not be present. Commonly, these symptoms are associated with falls.

To maintain normal balance, our inner ears, eyes, sense of position and cerebellum must all work together in an integrated fashion. Ageing is associated with degeneration of the inner ear apparatus and the cerebellum. There is also a reduced sense of position and poorer eyesight in the elderly. These factors contribute to the dizziness and unsteadiness that elderly people with dysequilibrium of ageing may experience.

Treatment is directed at reversible causes, and this takes time. I referred Madam Lee for a cataract operation, which improved her eyesight. At the same time, she was referred to the physiotherapist for gait training. The use of a walking stick increased her confidence and enabled her to walk without fear of falling. Madam Lee also saw the occupational therapist who advised her family on ways to improve home safety so as to lessen the chances of falling. For example, they were advised to leave a night light on so that Madam Lee would be able to make her way to the toilet at night.

The use of medication is frequently not necessary and may even lead to undesirable side effects. Common side effects of medicine for giddiness include drowsiness, dry mouth, constipation and even parkinsonism (tremors and rigidity).

Counselling is also important. Over the one-year period in which she came to see me, I allowed her to 'unload' all her complaints and feelings about her condition, and then gently led her to accept the 'uncomfortable' sensation of dysequilibrium. I tried as far as possible to avoid prescribing medication because the effect would be minimal. There is no cure for dysequilibrium of ageing.

4

Feelings Of Gloom And Doom

Emotional Suffering

Depression is an emotional state characterised by feelings of gloom and inadequacy. A local study reported that 4.6 per cent of the elderly living in a certain community had depression.

It is important to recognise and treat depression because depression causes much emotional suffering for the victim. It also impedes the progress of patients undergoing rehabilitation and may terminate in suicide.

Fortunately, the majority of us will not suffer from depression when we grow old. Even if we do suffer from depression, there is hope because depression is a treatable illness.

A Story about a Patient with Depression

Mr Yeo, a 76-year-old Chinese man, came to see me about a month ago, because he had started behaving strangely, was forgetful and had a poor appetite. His family also noted that he was talking to himself and praying to the wall. He was irritable. His memory, especially of recent events, was poor. He needed to be prompted to take a bath, and would not eat unless he was reminded again and again.

He repeatedly said that his deceased parents had come to find him and had told him to follow them. He kept telling his family that he wanted to die. At times, he would burst into tears for no obvious reason. At their wits' end, his family finally had to arrange a consultation for him when he refused to eat or drink.

The first thing that struck me when he came in was that he looked frail and miserable. There was no eye contact, no smile, no acknowledgment, as he mumbled his answers to my questions. Other than being dehydrated, I could not find anything wrong after a physical examination. As he was not eating or drinking, I had to admit him for treatment and observation.

While in hospital, we rehydrated him with an intravenous drip infusion. More blood tests were done, and these were also normal. The medical and nursing staff noted that he was rather passive, lying in bed the whole day and refusing to do anything for himself. At night, he slept poorly, waking up in the middle of the night and tossing about in bed as though in deep thought.

During this period, I had to spend time with the family to educate them about the condition, and to find out if there had been any family or personal conflict that could cause depression. There had been none. Not surprisingly, when the diagnosis of depression was made, the family members were reluctant to accept it: "But we love him and give him everything he wants, how could he be depressed? What is he depressed about?"

Nevertheless, he was started on an antidepressant. Over a period of two weeks in hospital, he gradually started to improve. He could even manage a smile, a 'thank you', and was more willing to do things for himself. On discharge from hospital, he was eating well and was in a better mood. He also talked to the hospital staff and joked with his family members.

Causes

Theories on causes of depression abound, but unfortunately nobody knows the exact cause(s). Depression is probably caused by a combination of factors such as genetic predisposition, structural and chemical brain disorders, hormonal disorders and environmental circumstances. Some factors associated with depression are old age, ill-health, personality dysfunction, hospitalisation and staying in a nursing home. Women are more prone to suffer from depression.

Diagnosis

Depression in the elderly can be difficult to diagnose. The patient usually does not declare that he is depressed. Instead, more commonly, he will have multiple physical complaints or may even complain of poor memory. These physical complaints are usually vague, and are often related to pain — like body aches, headaches and stomach pains. It is difficult to localise the cause of the pain as well.

The process of translating psychological pain into bodily pain and discomfort is called 'somatisation'. This somatisation may be the older person's way of drawing attention to himself. It is this somatisation or 'atypical presentation' that confuses the diagnosis and makes management difficult.

At the same time, relatives may note a change in behaviour; the person may be withdrawn or easily agitated. On direct questioning, the depressed patient may admit to the following complaints: insomnia, listlessness, loss of interest in life, poor appetite, and the inability to concentrate. Some cases may not be apparent until after the patient has attempted suicide.

The Geriatric Depression Scale on page 43 is a questionnaire which can be used to screen a candidate for depression. It can be self-administered or administered by a second party.

Suicide Risk

Nearly 90 per cent of suicides in the elderly are associated with depressive illness. Therefore, it is important to assess the likelihood of suicide in depressed elderly people. The critical periods of risk for suicide are the first few hours after hospitalisation and the first few weeks after discharge. The rate of suicide increases with age, until extreme late life, and then drops. Other factors associated with increased risk of suicide are social isolation, alcoholism, drug addiction, unemployment, talk about suicide, previous suicidal attempts and physical ill health. Men are at greater risk.

A myth that the mere mention of suicide may provoke the act is unfounded. In fact, most patients are only too grateful to know that someone understands their inclination to inflict harm on themselves.

Treating Depression

Depressed people cannot be expected to 'snap out' of their depression on their own. They need help to get them out of their gloom. They may require one or more of the following:

- change in mindset/behaviour (psychotherapy)
- treatment with drugs (pharmacotherapy)
- electric shock (electroconvulsive therapy or ECT)
- family therapy
- spiritual counselling.

Psychotherapy is usually for milder forms of depression. It involves countering negative habits of thinking about oneself, one's environment and the future (cognitive therapy). It also uses the technique of rewarding pleasant mood states while 'punishing' unpleasant mood states (behavioural therapy). Psychotherapy is usually administered by psychiatrists and psychologists.

Studies have shown that depressed patients respond better to a combination of antidepressant drugs and psychotherapy, compared to psychotherapy on its own. In severe or non-responding cases, electroconvulsive therapy (ECT) may be effective. This is done by passing an electrical current through the brain to induce a fit (seizure). The procedure is usually recommended by the psychiatrist, and performed with the patient under light general anaesthesia.

The family plays a very important role in supporting the depressed elders at home. They provide the environment, the acceptance, the understanding and support needed for recovery. They are also the ones who are there with the patient to ensure compliance to medication as well as to report progress in terms of mood changes or undeclared thoughts of suicide.

The spiritual aspect of depression cannot be ignored. Priests or pastors may have to be called in to provide spiritual counselling.

Drug Treatment

Many types of medication are used to treat depression. These are called 'antidepressants'.

It is important to understand that antidepressants may take between four and eight weeks to be effective. Therefore, patients and caregivers should not be excessively worried if there seems to be no change in the patient's mood after a few days of treatment.

Antidepressants, like other forms of medication, are not devoid of side effects. Tricyclic antidepressants (such as dothiepin) may cause a drop in blood pressure or drowsiness, worsen eyesight (for example, cause glaucoma) and cause heart conditions, constipation and difficulty in passing urine. The newer selective serotonin reuptake inhibitors (like fluvoxamine) are safer. However, they may cause nausea, headache, insomnia or drowsiness and result in a low sodium level in the blood.

The patient should inform the doctor that he or she is on antidepressants so that the doctor will avoid prescribing any drug that may adversely interact with the antidepressant.

Responding to Treatment

Generally, one-third of depressed elders recover from depression

Antidepressants and their Possible Side Effects

Class of Antidepressant	Examples	Some Possible Side Effects
Tricyclic Antidepressants (TCA)	Amitriptyline Imipramine Dothiepin Clomipramine	Dry mouth Drowsiness Constipation Difficulty with urination Dizziness Blurred vision
Tetracyclic antidepressants	Mianserin Maprotiline	May suppress bone marrow Lightheadedness Dizziness Dry mouth Sedation and drowsiness Nausea and vomiting
Monoamine Oxidase Inhibitors	Moclobemide	Dry mouth Postural hypotension Constipation Interactions with food containing tyramine like cheese, beer, preserved meats. May induce hypertension
Selective Serotonin Reuptake Inhibitor (SSRI)	Fluvoxamine Fluoxetine Sertraline Paroxetine Citapolam	Nausea Vomiting Diarrhoea Insomnia Agitation

within one year, one-third do not recover, while one-third do recover but experience a relapse. Elders who suffer from significant physical illness and from more severe and prolonged depression have poorer outcomes and higher death rates. Depression is common among the elderly and should not be ignored or overlooked. Most of them can be relieved of their suffering, if not cured with treatment.

Where to Seek Help

Depression in an older person is best handled by the geriatrician or a psychiatrist who specialises in the care of older persons (or psycho-geriatrician).

Geriatric Depression Scale
(to be self-administered or administered by a second party)

1. Are you basically satisfied with your life?   Yes ❏   No ❏

2. Have you dropped many of your activities and interests?   Yes ❏   No ❏

3. Do you feel that your life is empty?   Yes ❏   No ❏

4. Do you often get bored?   Yes ❏   No ❏

5. Are you in good spirits most of the time?   Yes ❏   No ❏

6. Are you afraid something bad is going to happen to you?   Yes ❏   No ❏

7. Do you feel happy most of the time?   Yes ❏   No ❏

8. Do you often feel helpless?   Yes ❏   No ❏

9. Do you prefer to stay at home, rather than go out and do new things?   Yes ❏   No ❏

10. Do you feel that you have more problems with memory than most?   Yes ❏   No ❏

11. Do you think it is wonderful to be alive now?   Yes ❏   No ❏

12. Do you feel pretty worthless the way you are now?   Yes ❏   No ❏

13. Do you feel that you are full of energy?   Yes ❏   No ❏

14. Do you feel that your situation is helpless?   Yes ❏   No ❏

15. Do you think most people are better off than you are?   Yes ❏   No ❏

(Please tick answer)

Score: 1 point for 'Yes' in 2, 3, 4, 6, 8, 9, 10, 12, 14, 15.
1 point for 'No' in 1, 5, 7, 11, 13.

0–5 points: normal   **above 5 points:** suggests depression

5

Huffing And Puffing

Fitness and Breathlessness

Everyone experiences breathlessness at some time or other. At the end of a 2.4 km run, everyone, even fit and tough commando trainees, is breathless. No one complains about that because that is considered 'normal' and is 'expected'. As we age, however, the amount of physical work we can do before we become breathless gradually diminishes. This is related to the ageing process and is also dependent on our individual levels of physical fitness, and of course the presence or absence of disease.

In my practice as a geriatrician, I find that the more common causes of breathlessness among older persons are related to cardiopulmonary diseases, that is, heart and lung diseases.

The Abused Lungs

Mr Lim, aged 70, had been smoking since age 15, when he dropped out of school. He worked first as a labourer and then as a lorry driver. In those days, smoking was fashionable and it also kept him awake during his hours of long-distance driving. He retired at the age of 65, citing poor health as a reason, as he had started coughing intermittently. His cough produced phlegm and occasionally disturbed his sleep at night.

Gradually over the past two years, he had become breathless on exertion, and had given up climbing the overhead bridge to cross the road. He was also unable to walk up a slope without stopping to catch his breath. About one week prior to seeing me, his cough and phlegm production had increased, and he had begun to feel more breathless. He had also developed a fever.

When I saw him at my clinic, I found him breathing heavily, as though he were fighting for breath. Further examination showed that he wheezed whenever he breathed, and that he was also suffering from pneumonia.

Mr Lim had been smoking for about 55 years, and it was apparent that since the age of 65, he had been having lung problems which had become worse over the past two years. His lung condition subsequently predisposed him to pneumonia.

What Causes Breathlessness?

Is breathlessness part of ageing? After all, Mr Lim is already 70 years old. A normal ageing elder does not get out of breath during daily activities such as bathing, dressing or walking. Although his lungs may become stiffer and less efficient in the absorption of oxygen (because of the ageing process), it will not cause breathlessness. Breathlessness occurs only if the lungs have previously been damaged by disease or cigarette smoking.

In fact, lung disease caused by cigarette smoking is one of the most common reasons for hospital admissions among the elderly. The damage from cigarette smoking builds up over the years and is akin to taking a slow poison. It may seem a glamorous thing to smoke when one is young, but calamity catches up during old age. Some people do seem to escape many of the illnesses associated with smoking even though they smoke like chimneys, but these are exceptions rather than the rule.

When a 'COLD' Is Not a Cold

Cigarette smoke irritates the delicate lining of the airways. Mucus production is increased and the hair-cells lining the airways are damaged. As a result of increased mucus production, inflammation and contraction of the muscles in the airways result in the wheezing that can sometimes be heard by the smoker. With prolonged smoking over several years, the terminal airways are also destroyed and the lungs no longer function efficiently. Oxygen exchange is impaired and the person will experience breathlessness during exertion or rigorous activities.

Of course, as the disease progresses, even mild activities such as climbing a flight of stairs may become a chore. And during advanced stages of the disease, difficulty in breathing or dyspnoea may be present even when the patient is at rest. This condition is commonly referred to as 'chronic obstruction lung disease' (or COLD) by medical doctors. It is by no means a benign condition such as a common cold. In its late stages the damage is often irreversible.

The person who smokes is also prone to lung diseases other than COLD. He is at higher risk for developing infections of the lungs or pneumonia. Because prolonged smoking destroys the terminal airways, the lungs are also more likely to puncture spontaneously and leak air. This is known as pneumothorax or air in the chest cavity.

Both the conditions mentioned above will further limit the efficiency of the lungs and the person will feel very short of breath. Hospitalisation is usually needed. In the case of pneumonia, antibiotic therapy will be required; if the condition is serious, intravenous antibiotics will be used and the patient may even need to inhale additional oxygen via a mask. For air leaks, a tube has to be inserted through the chest wall to drain the air and allow the lungs to re-expand. The tube is usually removed after a few days.

A person with COLD is prone to developing heart failure. This is also known as *cor pulmonale*, a Latin term which means right-sided heart failure. When the terminal airways are damaged, the blood supply around the airways is also affected. The heart has to pump harder to push blood through the lungs to extract oxygen. This extra strain eventually causes the right side of the heart to fail. During the later stage, the left side of the heart is also impaired.

Other smoking-related illnesses include cancer, especially lung cancer. The most common cause of lung cancer is cigarette smoking. Lung cancer may cause breathlessness and cough because it either obstructs the airways or causes fluid accumulation in the chest cavity. The latter condition is known medically as pleural effusion. Lung cancer is usually without symptoms during its early stage and by the time it causes respiratory symptoms, the tumour is usually large.

Some patients are fearful of seeing the doctor because they do not want to be confronted with such a diagnosis. Unfortunately, by the time they present themselves to the doctor, the cancer is at an advanced stage. It is important to consult the doctor early if you experience a chronic cough persisting over a month, or increasing breathlessness, or weight loss if you are a smoker. These symptoms could be a warning sign of lung cancer.

I started Mr Lim on oxygen therapy to help relieve his breathlessness. He was given antibiotics as well as bronchodilators, or drugs which open up the airways in the lungs. I also prescribed a course of chest physiotherapy to get rid of the excess mucus or phlegm. When his condition stabilised, I sat down with him to talk about quitting smoking!

Is It too Late to Quit Smoking?

Some smokers may argue that it is difficult to give up after so many years. Others will say that since the damage is already done, it is better to die happy with a cigarette in the mouth than to be deprived of cigarettes and be miserable for the rest of their lives. There is nothing further from the truth. Studies have now shown that once the damaging effects of cigarette smoking are removed, and the lungs are given a chance to recover, the damage can be reversed thus:

- within **8 hours** of the last cigarette smoked, the carbon monoxide level in the blood drops to normal while the oxygen level rises to normal
- after **72 hours**, the bronchial tubes relax, making breathing easier as the lung capacity increases
- after **2 weeks to 3 months**, lung function increases by one-third
- after **1 to 9 months**, coughing, sinus congestion, fatigue and shortness of breath are decreased, and cilia (hair cells) grow back in the lining of the bronchial tubes, increasing the ability to clear mucus and reduce infection
- after **5 years**, the lung cancer death rate decreases
- after **10 years**, the lung cancer death rate is almost the same as that of nonsmokers. Of course, the earlier cigarette smoking is stopped, the better. Less improvement is expected if smoking is given up only during the terminal stages of COLD.

Apart from the 'lung' benefits, giving up smoking also reduces high blood pressure and the risk of heart attacks, and improves fertility as well.

Quitting Smoking — an Uphill Task

It is never easy to quit when you have been smoking for the past 55 years, especially since smoking is addictive. Hence, I referred Mr Lim to a professional smoking cessation service. There are several agencies that provide such services. Appointments are required and there is usually a charge for the sessions, which may be held individually or in groups.

The Failing Heart

Seventy-year-old Mr Chua has been suffering from high blood pressure for more than 15 years. He sees his general practitioner periodically for tablets but has been irregular about treatment. He finds it a nuisance to take tablets daily as he feels fine on most days. However, one afternoon, he noticed that he was not as energetic as before and could not climb the four flights of steps to his flat without panting and perspiring profusely.

This observation, on top of the splitting headaches he had suffered lately, made him very worried and he decided to see his doctor the very same day. At the clinic, the doctor found that his blood pressure was extremely high — 230/110 mmHg. He was immediately referred for admission at the hospital where I have a practice.

He landed up in my ward, and by the time I saw him, he was lying breathless in bed. Clinical examination showed that Mr Chua had the symptoms of heart failure: congested neck veins, swelling of both feet, a fast heartbeat and congested lungs. His blood pressure was 220/115 mmHg. I made a diagnosis of heart failure caused by severe high blood pressure.

High Blood Pressure — another Silent Killer

High blood pressure or hypertension usually occurs without symptoms. Occasionally, it may give rise to headaches. Most cases of hypertension do not have known causes, and treatment therefore has to be lifelong. For these reasons, most hypertension patients are sometimes reluctant to take their medication regularly. They feel well and do not want to be bothered with their tablets. However, hypertension is not a benign disease, and if left untreated or inadequately treated for several years, may result in heart disease, stroke or kidney disease.

The elevated blood pressure places a strain on the heart, which has to pump harder to circulate the blood around the body.

The heart often compensates by enlarging its muscle mass to cope with the extra demand. However, there is a limit to the body's balancing act. With time, the heart may tire out and start to fail. Worse still, the blood vessels supplying the heart muscles and the coronary arteries may also be compromised and the patient may end up with a major heart attack or myocardial infarction. (See page 90.)

I started Mr Chua on diuretics and antihypertensive therapy. Diuretics are drugs which cause the body to lose water, thereby reducing the load on the failing heart. Examples of diuretics are frusemide (like Lasix) and bumetanide (like Burinex). When the condition is acute, diuretics may be given as intravenous injections, but once the fluid retention is under control, they can be taken orally.

Since the object is to reduce the load on the heart, in addition to increasing water loss through diuretics, the intake of salt (sodium) and water should also be restricted. Salt tends to retain water. Water intake should initially be restricted to less than a litre a day, then adjusted accordingly.

There are several types of antihypertensive agents which act on different sites. They are:

- diuretics which reduce blood pressure by reducing the load on the heart (e.g., hydrochlorothiazide);
- calcium channel blockers (e.g., nifedipine), ACE-inhibitors (e.g., captopril, enalapril) and alpha-adrenoceptor blockers (e.g., prazosin) which relax the blood vessel walls
- beta-blockers which reduce the heart rate and the strength of contraction of heart muscles (e.g., atenolol, propranolol), and
- clonidine and methyldopa, which act centrally in the brain to reduce blood pressure.

Centrally acting anti-hypertensives are less favoured as they have more side effects. The choice of drug is a matter of clinical judgement.

As Mr Chua's blood pressure came under control and his heart condition improved, so did his breathlessness. However, he must remember that hypertension is another silent killer, and not wait for symptoms to appear before he takes his medication.

Smoking Cessation Services in Singapore

1. **Child Guidance Clinic, Institute of Health**
   Telephone: 5345366. For students below age 18.

2. **Department of Psychology, Institute of Mental Health**
   Telephone: 3892126

3. **Singapore Cancer Society**
   Telephone: 4215806

4. **Stay Well Centre, Institute of Health**
   Telephone: 4353729

5. **Tampines Polyclinic**
   Telephone: 7864070

6. **Toa Payoh Polyclinic**
   Telephone: 2596833 ext 71

7. **Bukit Batok Polyclinic**
   Telephone: 5664583

8. **Youngberg Wellness Centre**
   Telephone: 2561055, 5660229

9. **Ang Mo Kio Acupuncture Research Clinic**
   Telephone: 4506712

6

Losing Control Of Bladder
And Bowels

Can Nothing Be Done?

Do you believe that when a person grows old, it is normal to lose
control of urinary or bowel movements? Have you heard from
your friends or relatives that nothing can be done when this
happens, because it is part of ageing? Well, many of my patients
and their relatives believed that. Do you?

Urinary Incontinence and the Causes

Urinary incontinence is the involuntary leakage of urine. The
sufferer is unable to control the bladder so that urine leaks out
and soils the clothing, linen or floor. The myth that urinary incontinence is part of growing old (erroneously called second child-
hood) must be dispelled.

Although it is more common in the older person (1 in 10 of
them), urinary incontinence is abnormal, unless you are a baby.
In other words, all of us are born incontinent! In Singapore, about
15 per cent of people above age 60 and living at home have
urinary incontinence. This percentage goes up in the hospitals
and among those in nursing homes.

The common causes vary depending on age:

- Bedwetting at night (or enuresis) in the 5 to 15 age group is usually due to delayed maturation of the brain's control of the bladder function. It is associated with a strong family history of enuresis and is more common in boys.

- In the 15 to 25 age group, poor bladder habits resulting in an irritable bladder or injuries to the spine affecting the nerves serving the bladder and the sphincters (muscles around the outlet of the bladder) are the usual causes.

- When it comes to the 25 to 50 age group, the most common cause in women is weak pelvic floor muscles, while in men it is usually due to an irritable bladder.

- With the 50 to 75 age group, urinary infection and menopause are common causes in women, while enlarged prostate is the usual culprit in men.

- In the 'old-old' age group (over 75 years), incontinence is usually caused by a combination of factors: aggravation of the preexisting incontinence problems mentioned, poor physical or mental state, adverse effects of medication and poor environmental conditions.

We must always remember that urinary incontinence is merely a symptom or a sign of an underlying problem, just like fever and cough. We must search for the underlying cause, and not stop at treating the symptom.

Together with Staff Nurse Tan, a continence nurse advisor (a state-registered nurse trained specially in the management of incontinence), I run a continence clinic at the hospital where I practise. At this clinic, we see many patients with various causes of incontinence. Some are treated and healed completely, while in others, the incontinence is controlled.

The Infected Bladder

Madam Siva, a 71-year-old Indian, was referred to the continence clinic because her family noticed that she had begun to smell of urine. For almost three weeks she had leaked urine, sometimes onto the toilet floor, but often on her underpants before she could reach the toilet. She had to rush to the toilet very frequently.

Although she felt some pain in her lower abdomen each time she passed urine, she denied having a burning sensation (commonly present in those with urinary infection). She did not complain of fever, and was able to carry out her daily housework. She has hypertension and diabetes, and has been taking her medication regularly.

I proceeded to examine her, in particular to see if there was any tenderness or distension of the bladder that would suggest that Madam Siva was not able to empty her bladder completely. I found that there was no redness or soreness of her genitalia that might indicate persistent wetting, poor hygiene, infection or atrophic vaginitis (dryness of the vagina from inadequate estrogen hormone).

Next, I inserted a finger into her anus to examine her rectum (the part of the intestine where stools are stored). This procedure, called a rectal examination, was done to ensure that she was not constipated. A grossly distended rectum (from constipation) may irritate the bladder to give the same symptoms that Madam Siva had complained about.

I then checked her blood glucose level as she was diabetic. This is because when the blood glucose is high, it causes an increase in urine production, and the affected person has to rush to the toilet frequently and urgently to pass urine. Poor control would also predispose the person to infection.

The result of the urine test confirmed my initial suspicion: there was an abnormal number of pus cells in the urine sample.

This indicated that she had urinary infection. The infection had irritated the bladder to give her the sensation of pain and discomfort in her lower abdomen, as well as the frequency and urgency that resulted in the leakage of urine.

I gave her a course of antibiotics, and advised her to drink at least 1,500 ml of water daily. This was to ensure that she had a regular flow of urine to 'flush' out the bladder. A week later, Madam Siva returned for a review. She was cured.

The 'Unstable' Bladder

Another important and common cause of urinary incontinence in the elderly is the 'unstable' bladder. Although the true rate of incidence of this condition is not known, it is more common with advancing age, neurological diseases and enlargement of the prostate gland (in men). The affected persons have the urge to pass urine frequently and quickly. Leakage of urine occurs because they cannot reach the toilet in time. This is known as urge urinary incontinence.

At age 78, Madam Wu had been well until last October when she suffered a stroke resulting in weakness of the left side of her body. After her discharge from hospital, her daughter noticed that she was always asking to go to the toilet to pass urine. Each time she went there, she would pass only 'a few drops' of urine. She would also leak urine when she was not attended to immediately. Her daughter became tired of assisting her to the toilet. She interpreted this as a 'cry wolf' or 'attention-seeking' ploy on her mother's part.

After a thorough examination, I tested Madam Wu's urine for infection but it was clear. She opened her bowels regularly, and the rectal examination was normal. I advised her daughter to do a bladder chart to monitor her mother's urinary habits. This chart would give objective evidence of the severity of her urinary problem, and also help to monitor her progress. She was

BLADDER CHART

Instructions:
(1) Record the quantity of each fluid intake and the time it was taken.
(2) Record the time urine was passed and the amount produced.
(3) If the quantity of fluid or urine is not known, please make a tick.
(4) Under remarks, record events that may explain wetting or discrepancies in the charting, like urinal spilled, used diapers, passed into toilet.

DATE: DATE:

TIME	INTAKE (in ml)	AMOUNT VOIDED (in ml)	REMARKS	TIME	INTAKE (in ml)	AMOUNT VOIDED (in ml)	REMARKS

required to chart the time of day and amount of urine passed over three consecutive days. Indeed, the chart showed that she passed only a small amount of urine each time (between 5 ml and 30 ml), 25 times during the day and seven times after going to bed at night. No wonder the daughter got terribly tired of her repeated requests to be taken to the toilet!

To make sure that she was emptying her bladder adequately, I did a bladder scan after she had passed urine. This is an important test because inadequate emptying (either from weakness of the bladder wall muscles or from obstruction at the bladder outlet) should be treated promptly to prevent potential complications like recurrent infections and damage to the kidneys. Moreover, in cases such as Madam Wu's, where there is inadequate emptying of the bladder, the bladder fills up quickly, giving rise to the complaint of too-frequent urination.

Madam Wu's bladder scan was normal. Since her urinary problem came on soon after a stroke, and there were no other conditions (like urinary infection) that could cause the symptoms, I diagnosed Madam Wu to be suffering from an unstable bladder.

In a normal person, nerves from the bladder will inform the brain about fullness of the bladder. Nerves from the brain to the bladder (facilitatory nerves) will either facilitate bladder contraction, resulting in voiding; or relax the bladder (inhibitory nerves) so that it can continue to hold the urine. This gives the person voluntary control over when he or she decides to void. A number of neurological conditions like Parkinson's Disease and spinal cord injury affect this fine balance; in Madam Wu's case, a stroke had been the cause.

Bladder Re-Education

I asked Nurse Tan to teach Madam Wu how to overcome the urge to pass urine. She was taught to tighten her pelvic floor muscles (muscles around her anus, vagina and urethra) for about

10 seconds, take a few deep breaths, and focus her mind on something pleasant. She was to repeat the process each time she had the urge to pass urine. Meanwhile, she was allowed to pass urine in the bedpan or toilet only at the scheduled time. Although she might leak initially, this would improve over time. This process of training is called bladder re-education.

I also prescribed a small dose of anticholinergic drug (like oxybutinin) that might help to relax the bladder. Nurse Tan also explained Madam Wu's condition to her daughter, and stressed the need for her to enforce the training regime diligently at home. Although bladder re-education cannot cure the bladder condition, improvement following such treatment may be apparent as early as at the end of the first week. A period of up to three months is usually needed to regain full control.

By the next visit, the daughter was certainly happier. The bladder chart showed a vast improvement: Madam Wu had passed urine only about six times during the day, once at night, and she wetted herself only occasionally. She had also regained enough confidence in her bladder to go shopping, albeit in a wheelchair.

The Leaky Bladder

Another common complaint among sufferers of urinary incontinence, especially women, is that they leak urine when they cough, sneeze, laugh, jump, or lift something heavy. This is known as stress urinary incontinence, and is often caused by weak pelvic floor muscles. The weakness is usually a consequence of difficult childbirth, insufficient care and exercise after delivery of babies, damage to nerves supplying the pelvic floor muscles, or constant straining on passing out stools. In severe cases of weak pelvic floor muscles, the person may leak urine on standing up or walking, and at times even while sleeping, when the bladder is full.

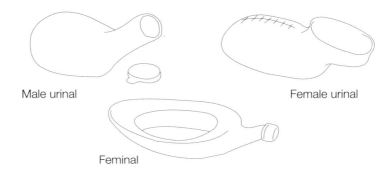

Male urinal   Female urinal

Feminal

Bedpans and and urinals are handy aids for
incontinent, bedridden elderly persons.

Madam Koh, 76, saw me because she leaked urine every time she sneezed. This problem had been going on for some years, but was aggravated recently because she came down with influenza. She is obese and has five children, all of whom had been big babies. She had also had a difficult forceps delivery for her last baby.

The best treatment for weak pelvic floor muscles are pelvic floor exercises (PFE). I asked Nurse Tan to show Madam Koh where her pelvic floor muscles are, and to show her how the exercises are done. As her condition was mild, nothing more needed was required except to advise her to lose weight and continue with PFE, which when done diligently could achieve improvement within six weeks.

In some cases of stress urinary incontinence, electrical stimulation and estrogen therapy are useful in addition to PFE. Electrical stimulation helps to prime the pelvic floor muscles further and augment the regular PFE. Estrogens (applied topically as a cream, or in pessary or 'tablet' form) may help if there is evidence of atrophic vaginitis. Finally, in severe cases, surgery to repair the weak pelvic floor or to tighten the outlet may be useful.

The Atonic (Flaccid) Bladder

Mr Arnie Lee is one of the unlucky few who has a disorder of the bladder that cannot be cured. Despite this, he has been able to remain continent and in control of his bladder. Arnie, 46, was a successful businessman holidaying in New Guinea when the tour bus he was in overturned while negotiating a bend. When he woke up, he found that he was paralysed from the waist downwards and had a tube draining urine (indwelling catheter) from his bladder. He had lost awareness and control of his bladder as his spinal cord had been damaged in the accident.

The initial shock was most distressing and unbearable, but with lots of encouragement and support from his family, nurses and doctors, he quickly regained his composure. He vowed to function as normally as possible for someone who would be permanently chairbound.

Soon after his return to Singapore, he saw me and asked if the indwelling catheter could be removed. It was uncomfortable, unsightly, and what was more, he was getting repeated urinary infections from it. I did a urodynamic study to check on the state of the bladder. This is a study where small tubes are inserted into the bladder, one to fill it, the other to measure the pressure generated by the bladder. The study confirmed that he had an atonic or flaccid bladder: he had no sensation of fullness of the bladder at all, and the bladder failed to contract even when distended to 600 ml (normal bladder capacity is about 500 ml).

He would require artificial drainage of urine from his bladder permanently. One way of doing this is to drain the bladder with an indwelling urinary catheter; that is, the catheter is left in place in the bladder with the outer free end connected to a urine bag. This is usually done at the expense of frequent urinary infections, which Arnie was already experiencing. A better method is to do 'clean, intermittent self-catheterisation' (CISC).

Do-It-Yourself Catheter Care

For Men

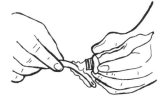

1. Lubricate the catheter.

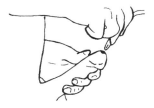

2. Insert the catheter.

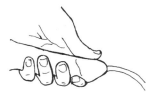

3. Urinate.

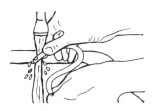

4. Wash the catheter.

For Women

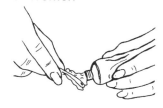

1. Lubricate the catheter.

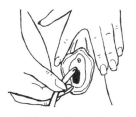

2. Insert the catheter.

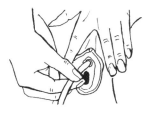

3. Urinate.

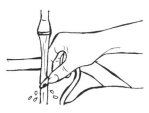

4. Wash the catheter.

Clean Intermittent Catheterisation

CISC is done by introducing a tube into the person's own urethra (passage for urine to come out) at six-hourly intervals to drain the urine completely. In this way, the bladder will not be over-distended, and there is no accumulation of stagnant urine or a foreign body (like an indwelling catheter) that predisposes the urinary tract to infection. Although his bladder may be paralysed and will never recover, Arnie is still in control over a part of his bladder function: to store urine until he is ready to empty it, without any leakage or incontinence in between.

While Arnie may be young (in his late 40s), many older folks with similar problems can undergo a similar treatment procedure with slight variations. Older folks with poor coordination and weak hands will need someone to catheterise them. This process is known as 'clean intermittent catheterisation by caregivers' (CICC). The procedure must be properly taught by the continence nurse advisor who will also provide written guidelines for the caregivers' reference, until they are familiar with it.

Intermittent catheterisation is a very suitable technique for treating someone who is unable to empty the bladder effectively. It prevents the complications of ineffective emptying such as repeated episodes of urinary infection, overflow incontinence, or in some cases, kidney failure.

Common causes of ineffective emptying of the bladder in the elderly are complications of diabetes mellitus and damage of bladder muscles due to chronic over-distension, a frequent occurrence in those with stroke, enlarged prostate gland or constipation. Adverse effects of certain medications and failure to detect such problems early often aggravate the condition.

Protecting your Bladder

Can urinary incontinence be prevented? Except for cases with congenital causes, urinary incontinence may be prevented. The following guidelines are useful in keeping the bladder healthy:

1. Drink at least 1.5 litres of fluid per day, unless advised otherwise by your doctor.

2. Limit the amount of caffeine and alcohol intake. Drink less coffee, tea or cola.

3. Practise good toilet habits: do not go to the toilet 'just in case'; go only when the bladder is full. You can check the amount you void to confirm that it is full. (Each void should be between 250 ml and 500 ml.) However, it is normal to empty your bladder before going to bed.

4. Take your time when urinating to ensure that your bladder empties completely.

5. Maintain good bowel habits and avoid persistent straining at stools. See 'Healthy Habits for Preventing Constipation' on page 71.

6. Do pelvic floor exercises regularly.

Seek help early if you have warning signs of bladder problems. The warning signs are explained on page 72.

Bowel Incontinence

Mr TMS, an 82-year-old Filipino, tried desperately to make an appointment at the Geriatric Centre to see the doctor as soon as possible. He claimed that he had frequent diarrhoea and did not wish to elaborate further. When I saw him, he revealed that he was passing motion frequently and it was so bad that he had been staining his trousers for the past 10 days. He felt very embarrassed when his other three roommates kept inquiring why he had to change and wash so frequently.

His problem started two weeks before when he had influenza. He had taken some medication for a running nose, sneezing and an irritating cough. His bowel habits subsequently became irregular and infrequent. He passed small amounts of watery stools, often with difficulty. In spite of moving his bowels so frequently, he felt that he had not emptied his bowels completely. The final straw came when he started soiling his underwear at least three or four times daily.

When I examined him, I noted that his abdomen was slightly distended. His underwear was also stained with stools. A rectal examination confirmed my suspicion: the anus and rectum were loaded with hard stools.

When I told Mr TMS that his problem was due to constipation, he was confused.

"Doctor, are you sure? I am having such bad diarrhoea that it has soiled my underwear. Don't tell me you're going to give me laxatives to make things worse!" He had wanted me to prescribe some anti-diarrhoea medicine instead.

I had to explain to him that he was suffering from 'spurious' diarrhoea. It is diarrhoea that is caused by constipation. As a result of constipation, the stools stored in the rectum become dry, and so shrink in size. Over time, they become hard like pellets, and are packed tightly into one another. In severe cases, they distend the rectum and the anal sphincters as well. These hard pellets of stools irritate the rectal wall, causing the rectum to secrete mucus. When it comes in contact with the stools, the mucus becomes stained, and being watery, leaks from the distended anal sphincter. This soiling is called faecal incontinence.

Having understood why I had diagnosed constipation instead of diarrhoea, he was willing to have an enema (washout to empty the rectum), as well as to take the laxatives until his bowel habits returned to normal. By the time he returned in a fortnight, he was cured.

Mr TMS is among the four per cent of elderly in the community with faecal incontinence. In nursing homes, 10 per cent may have the problem. Almost 14 per cent of admissions (of those above age 65) to one geriatric ward in Singapore in 1994 had this problem. It is important to note that faecal incontinence is not a consequence of old age.

Mr TMS had regular, daily bowel movements before his attack of influenza. It was neither that nor his age that had caused him to have faecal incontinence; the side effects of the cough syrup and tablets for his running nose had led to constipation and subsequently faecal incontinence. Other common drugs that have a constipating side effect include antacids containing aluminum, blood pressure pills like calcium channel blockers, painkillers containing codeine or opoids, sedatives and iron tablets.

Other factors that contribute to constipation include the lack of physical mobility and inadequate intake of fluids and fibre. Other causes of constipation include disorders like a low thyroid hormone state, high levels of calcium electrolyte in the blood, spinal cord injury and cancer of the colon. In many individuals, the cause of constipation is not known but habitual postponement in answering the need to move the bowels since young or chronic laxative abuse are implicated.

Besides constipation, faecal incontinence may be a symptom of underlying diseases of the colon such as cancer, diverticular disease and inflammatory bowel disease, or of severe diarrhoea from food poisoning. Diverticular disease is a common condition of the colon. It is characterised by multiple 'finger-like' projections extending from the lumen, or cavity of the colon, into the wall of the colon.

Faecal incontinence is also seen in patients with dementia from Alzheimer's Disease or multiple stroke disease. They have regular bowel movements but are unable to inhibit their urge to defecate. Some are unable to indicate their need to move their bowels.

Severe faecal incontinence is seen in those with failure of the anal sphincter. In such patients, they soil their underwear frequently because their anal sphincter is weak. Implicated causes include frequent straining at defecation, difficult childbearing, the use of surgical instruments during childbirth, and damage to the sphincter following surgery for piles.

The elderly sometimes suffer from faecal incontinence because they are unable to have access to a toilet or have difficulty unfastening their clothing. This situation occurs particularly in institutions like hospitals or nursing homes where shorthanded staff are unable to attend to these elderly promptly.

Prevention of Faecal Incontinence and the Use of Laxatives

Treating and preventing constipation are among the best strategies to reduce the risk of both faecal and urinary incontinence. There are a number of procedures for treating and preventing constipation. See 'Healthy Habits for Preventing Constipation' on page 71.

Laxatives are probably the most thoughtlessly prescribed drugs, be they self-prescribed or prescribed by the doctor. Chronic laxative abuse aggravates constipation. Other adverse effects include flatulence, abdominal discomfort or cramps, and malabsorption of vitamins A, D, E and K. A good understanding of the various modes of action of different laxatives, coupled with proper guidance from the physician, will help one to be more rational in the proper use of laxatives. There are four main groups of laxatives: bulk-forming agents, stimulant or irritant laxatives, osmotic laxatives and stool softeners.

Fibres are bulk-forming agents which relieve constipation after a few days by increasing faecal mass that stimulates bowel movements. One must take a sufficient quantity of fluids to prevent the formation of hard stools. They are not recommended for those who are bedbound. Wheat and oat bran are natural sources of fibre. Commercially available agents (for example,

Fybogel and Metamucil) contain ispaghula husk, methycellulose or sterculia.

Stimulant laxatives like Senna and Dulcolax increase intestinal motility, but prolonged use is associated with an atonic non-functioning colon. They are usually taken before bedtime as their action starts about 8 to 12 hours after consumption. The suppository form of Dulcolax works within one hour.

Osmotic laxatives (for example, Lactulose) increase faecal weight, volume and water content. Doses of more than 20 ml twice daily may be required.

Stool softeners such as liquid paraffin are usually to be avoided by the elderly because of the risk of inhalation pneumonia and interference with absorption of vitamins A, D, E and K.

Most suppositories (such as Glycerol and Dulcolax) and enemas (for example, Micralax and Fleet) are local irritants and dosage should be limited to not more than thrice weekly. They are useful for clearing faecal loading.

Treatment Strategies for Faecal Incontinence

Another common strategy for treating faecal incontinence is to strengthen the sphincter and the muscles supporting it with pelvic floor exercises, a strategy used also in the treatment of urinary stress incontinence. This is particularly successful in the very motivated with impaired sphincter following traumatic childbirth or those who had babies removed with surgical instruments. Surgical repair of the sphincter may be needed in those cases with severe damage.

Treatment that involves establishing a regular toilet routine is especially useful for those with dementia or those who do not have ready access to toilet facilities. It is preferable to go to the toilet after a meal to take advantage of the increase in intestinal activity. In the initial stage, the habit may be enhanced with judicious short-term use of laxatives.

When all treatment strategies fail to control faecal incontinence, a regimen combining constipation and anti-diarrhoea agents and planned evacuation with laxatives at regular intervals can be instituted. Get the proper advice from your doctor or the continence nurse advisor.

Importance of Proper Evaluation

Once again, I want to highlight the fact that faecal incontinence and constipation should not be regarded as an inevitable consequence of old age. Every attempt should be made to identify and correct reversible factors. Our next patient, Mr Tan, will further illustrate the importance of proper evaluation and correct treatment in curing his dual problems of urinary and bowel incontinence.

Mr Tan, 72, enjoys good food and has been treated for gout for many years. He is otherwise healthy. Trouble began 18 months ago when he started to open his bowels more often than usual, about two to three times daily. He thought that the cause might be old age, and perhaps that the Chinese tea that he had gulped in large quantities for many years might be too cooling for him.

When there was no improvement after three months, he told his daughter about it. She, in turn, thought that it might be the bread he had been eating that had caused it. She had been preparing high fibre bread with *kaya* (coconut jam) for his afternoon tea. It could be the fibre or perhaps a mild degree of food poisoning, since the *kaya* at room temperature might attract bacteria, she reasoned. As there was no diarrhoea, mucus or blood in the stools, and he did not have to wake up at night to move his bowels, it was probably not significant, she thought. After all, she was a staff nurse of many years' experience.

She decided to get cultured milk drinks for Mr Tan. This was supposed to increase the good bacteria in the intestines. After trying that for three months, the diarrhoea became worse. Not only had it become more frequent (up to five times daily), he had to rush to the toilet because the stools would very quickly find their way out. He had to ensure that he was out of the house only for short periods, and he would try to clear his bowels before he left.

When his married son, who happens to be a doctor, came to know about it, he suggested that the father go for a colonoscopy (a procedure where a tube with a viewing mirror is passed into the intestines). Mr Tan, however, preferred to continue seeing the *sinseh* (Chinese doctor) as he did not like the idea of having tubes put into his body. He had a few courses of both pills and mixtures, which appeared to work. The stools had remained pasty, but at times he would only need to visit the toilet three to four times a day.

Another five months passed and the problem returned and became worse. He had to visit the toilet almost immediately after a meal. He seemed to have lost control of his bowels, because whenever he passed urine, a small amount of stools would come out at the same time. When he thought that he wanted only to pass gas, some liquid stools would emerge as well. His urinary habits had also become abnormal. He had to visit the toilet often (once every one to two hours) and had to wake up two to three times at night. He had to strain to get his urine out, often aggravating the leakage of stools.

At times, the urgency to pass urine was so overwhelming that he would wet his trousers even before he could reach the toilet. He dared not go out of the house and was terribly upset that he had lost control of both his bladder and bowel movements. Finally, he agreed to go for tests.

A colonoscopy was done. It revealed a 6 cm cancerous growth in the rectum about 8 cm from the anal opening. Mr Tan went through a six-hour operation to have the growth removed. The growth had stuck to the sacral wall because of the formation of pus from a leak in the growth. It had lifted the bladder upwards. No wonder Mr Tan had to pass urine many times and had difficulty in clearing the urine each time.

Following surgery, his urinary habits gradually returned to normal. With an increase in dietary fibre to ensure that his stools were well formed, and pelvic floor exercises to strengthen his anal sphincter, Mr Tan managed to regain full control of his bowel and bladder movements three months after surgery. He has found a new pastime — window shopping in big shopping complexes.

Conclusion

It is never normal to lose control of your urinary or bowel movements. Even if a cure is not possible (which is likely to be the case if the cause is not known or detected too late), improvement in the condition and help for both the sufferer and the caregiver is always possible. If you have noticed in anyone a change in urinary or bowel habits that cannot be explained, or been told of such a change by someone who has experienced abnormality in urinary or bowel movements, do get that person to consult a doctor or get an appointment to see the continence nurse advisor. This advisor is stationed at any of the continence clinics listed on page 72.

Healthy Habits for Preventing Constipation

1. Drink at least 1.5 litres of water per day (unless otherwise advised by the doctor).

2. Increase daily dietary fibre intake to 20 g (unless bedbound).

3. Exercise daily, including plenty of walking (a minimum of 20 minutes, twice daily).

4. Develop a regular toilet routine:

   - Go to the toilet at the same time every day, preferably 15–30 minutes after a meal taken with an extra glass of warm water.

   - Sit comfortably and relax. Massage the abdomen gently in a circular movement — from right to left, and up and down — several times. Strain gently only when the urge is felt.

   - If no urge is felt after 10 minutes, stimulate the back passage (anus) by placing your hand on it and pushing upwards with the flat of your fingers. Let them remain still for five seconds, and then let go for five seconds. Repeat these actions for up to five minutes. You may protect your fingers with toilet paper. If no urge is felt after a further five minutes, abandon the toilet. Return to the toilet only when the urge is felt.

5. Take two tablets of Senna at night before going to bed on the day when there is no bowel movement, and on the third day of constipation, do the following:

   - Insert the prescribed suppository into the anus and return to the toilet when the urge is felt (usually 30–60 minutes later).

   - If bowel movement does not occur one hour after the suppository is inserted, give the recommended enema thus: insert the opening of the tube gently into the anus and squeeze the contents towards the back. Bowel movement should occur within the next 30 minutes.

6. Seek medical help early if any unexpected problems arise.

Warning Signs of Bladder Problems

1. Any involuntary leakage of urine, regardless of the amount (unless it happens to someone younger than age 5).

2. Urgent need to pass urine or to rush to the toilet.

3. Passing urine frequently (more than eight times per day) or small amounts each time (less than 200 ml).

4. Having to get up more than twice at night to pass urine.

5. Difficulty getting a stream of urine started or if the stream stops and starts instead of flowing out smoothly.

6. Having to strain to pass urine.

7. A sense that the bladder is not empty, despite having just passed urine.

8. A sensation of burning or discomfort while passing urine.

9. Passing blood or cloudy urine.

10. Any change in the regular urinary or bladder voiding pattern that is causing concern.

Continence Clinics in Singapore

1. **Alexandra Geriatric Centre.** Telephone: 4708415.

2. **Changi General Hospital.** Telephone: 8502580.

3. **Tan Tock Seng Hospital.** Telephone: 3595048.

4. **Ang Mo Kio Senior Citizens' Health Care Centre (SCHCC).** Telephone: 4506150.

5. **Bukit Batok SCHCC.** Telephone: 5634476.

6. **Geylang East SCHCC.** Telephone: 7468671.

7. **Hougang SCHCC.** Telephone: 3820274.

8. **Toa Payoh SCHCC.** Telephone: 2590669.

9. **Tampines SCHCC.** Telephone: 7865373.

Eating Your Way To Health
Or Sickness

Getting the Right Diet

Singaporeans love to eat. Food is a source of pleasure but it should also provide nourishment. While good nutrition has been well emphasised in the growing years, much of what the older person should or should not eat is not so well known. Hence, in my experience, many have already formed their own views about food and nutrition.

I have met some who feel that the older person should take more salt to compensate for the lack of taste, or that they do not need so much protein, which is not well digested. Others have turned to vegetarian diets because 'such diets are more healthy'. There are also the extremists who not only take full meals, but also pop vitamin pills 'just to make sure'. The list goes on. So who is right?

The Story of Madam Lee

Eighty-eight-year-old Madam Lee lived alone in a one-room HDB flat. She had a son and an adopted daughter, and both lived a few blocks away. They visited her only once every two weeks because of their work and family commitments. After losing her teeth, Madam Lee had had difficulty getting a well-fit set of dentures, so she had been eating porridge.

She also had a chronic heart and lung condition, and some of her medications were quite expensive. In order to save money for these, she cut back on her food. She took some minced meat and mashed vegetables only about once a week. She did not disclose this to her children as she did not want to worry or burden them further. They noticed she was getting weaker and losing weight, and bought some vitamin tablets for her. When these appeared not to help, they decided on a consultation.

When I saw Madam Lee, she was thin and frail. While standing 1.5 metres tall, she weighed only 34 kg. The facial muscles around her temples were wasted, and she looked pale and had mildly swollen feet. Her skin was coarse and dry, especially around the corners of the mouth. Her dentures appeared to be poorly fitted as they kept dropping off as she spoke. Subsequent blood tests showed that she was malnourished — she had anaemia, a low folic acid level and a very low protein (albumin) level which could account for her swollen feet.

Madam Lee's children had no idea of her difficulties. They had assumed that everything was fine because that was what she always said when they asked after her health. A better way of ensuring that she was eating properly would be to take a greater interest in her eating habits. I encouraged the children not only to question her, but also to check the refrigerator and to arrange regular shopping trips with her.

They could also enrol her on a meals-on-wheels programme (for those who have difficulty cooking for themselves) or simply organise a regular meal with a neighbour, relative or friend. It is always more enjoyable to eat with someone and socialise over a meal than to eat alone. Some senior citizens' centres also organise regular luncheons for old people living alone.

Malnutrition Defined

Malnutrition is caused by an excess, imbalance or deficit of nutrient(s) in relation to physiological needs. Factors that affect the adequacy of nutrient intake are mostly related to the quantity of food eaten. However, many people are unaware of what foods to choose or cannot afford food that is high in nutritional value. Hence, poor food selection can also lead to specific nutrient deficiencies.

The basic guidelines for a nutritious diet in the older person are the same for most healthy adults. Older people, however, need to pay special attention to the quality of food that they eat.

Calories and Fat

The older person needs fewer calories because of changes in the body and decreasing physical activity. This explains why many people gain weight more easily as they grow older. Limiting the amount of fat in the diet may help to prevent weight gain. Excess weight is associated with diabetes mellitus, heart disease and high blood pressure. Besides reducing the occurrence of these disorders, limiting the fat in the diet may also protect against some cancers.

Salt

As people grow older their sensitivity to flavour and smell often decreases. As a result, they may use more salt (usually sodium) to combat the 'flat' taste of food. However, older people should be cautious about using too much salt. Overuse is associated with high blood pressure. Restricting the amount of salt in the diet can control high blood pressure in many people who already have the disease.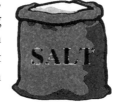

You can change a few dietary habits that will reduce the amount of salt without greatly changing the diet. Fresh foods have less salt than processed ones. Fresh meat has a lower salt content than bacon, hot dogs, sausages and ham, all of which

Salt Content of Some Common Food Items

Low Salt	High Salt
pork chop	bacon ham luncheon meat pork sausage
boiled egg	salted egg
powdered milk	cheddar cheese
cabbage	salted vegetables
boiled carrots	canned peas
potatoes	baked beans
peanut butter	canned chicken soup canned mushroom soup

use salt to flavour and preserve them. Likewise, most fresh vegetables naturally contain less salt than canned vegetables and vegetable juices, to which salt is usually added. Commercially prepared food such as soups, frozen dinners and other 'fast food' items have salt added during preparation. Snacks such as potato chips, corn chips, crackers and nuts normally have a lot of salt added to them, and are best eaten sparingly.

Vegetarianism

In general, vegetarians have a lower risk of obesity, hypertension, coronary heart disease and cancer of the large intestine. Does this mean that they are healthier than non-vegetarians?

Traditional vegetarianism has a long history, and as a result there exists a large number of healthy vegetarian dishes using ingredients rich in protein such as legumes and nuts. New vegetarians, however, especially those who simply remove meat from their diet, may be eating inadequately.

There are varying degrees of vegetarianism and each of them may have some nutritional risks:

1. Pecso-vegetarians are those who do not eat meat, but take fish, eggs and dairy products. They have very little nutritional risk.

2. Lacto-ovo-vegetarians avoid meat and fish, but take dairy products and eggs. This is the commonest form of vegetarianism. The potential nutritional risk is iron deficiency, as they miss 'haem' iron, the best form of iron in the diet. This group largely compensates with ascorbic acid (vitamin C), which enhances the absorption of non-haem iron.

3. Vegans do not eat any animal products—meat, fish, dairy products and eggs. They are therefore at high risk for Vitamin B_{12} deficiency. Adequate protein intake can be ensured if they regularly take leguminous products and nuts. Vegans also lack the best dietary sources of calcium. They should watch their intake of calcium, iron and zinc.

Vitamins and Minerals

"Vitamins are like seat belts. Wearing a seat belt doesn't give you a licence to drive recklessly, it just protects you in case of an accident. Vitamin supplements work in the same way; they don't give you a licence to eat poorly and otherwise abuse your health, but provide an added cushion of protection."

— P.J. Skerrett

Vitamins are organic compounds that are required in the diet for the maintenance of normal health. They are derived from animal or plant sources. Some are fat soluble, like vitamins A, D, E and K, and are stored in the body. The rest are water soluble, like vitamins B and C, and are generally not stored, but passed out in the urine. Minerals, on the other hand, are inorganic elements found in soil and water. Both vitamins and minerals are required by the body in small amounts and are abundant in fruit, meat, dairy products and whole grains.

"How else [other than taking vitamin supplements] can I be sure I'll get the right amount of vitamins in my diet?" you might ask. Unless you are under a doctor's care and eating less than 1,200 calories a day, or not eating a balanced diet, you need not worry about getting enough vitamins. Everything the body needs for good health is available in our natural food. However, since the body cannot store the B complex, it is essential that you eat a balanced diet every day to replenish this vitamin.

There is still little evidence to back most of these claims. Currently, many scientists are interested in 'free radicals'. They are believed to be responsible for much of the internal damage that accumulates over a lifetime, as well as some diseases that go with them. Free radicals are substances with unpaired electrons produced by the body's normal metabolism. Being 'charged particles', they latch on to various components of the cells in the body and damage them.

Recent studies have indicated that many diseases associated with ageing, including arthritis, cancer, cataracts, heart and lung diseases, osteoporosis, degeneration of the nervous system and a failing immune system may be due to free radicals.

Certain vitamins may be able to halt or even reverse these diseases. Much of this research has focused on the antioxidant role of vitamins C, E and beta-carotene (which the body converts to vitamin A) and the mineral selenium. Antioxidants neutralise free radicals by pairing up with their electrons. Antioxidants are present in most fruits, vegetables and whole grains. Enriching your diet with natural sources of antioxidants may boost your body's fight against free radicals.

If a little is Good, then is a lot Better?

Too often, people take high-dose supplements of various vitamins and minerals without a doctor's advice. The use of megavitamins and high potency formulae are of concern. These supplements contain 10 to 100 times the recommended daily allowance (RDA). People take them because they think that RDAs are only minimum requirements and that if a little is good, then surely a lot must be better.

This can be a waste of money or worse, a threat to health. Large amounts of vitamin A or D are particularly dangerous. Too much vitamin A can cause headaches, nausea, diarrhoea and eventually liver and bone damage. High doses of vitamin D cause kidney damage and even death. When taken in excessive amounts, supplemental iron can build up to harmful levels in the liver and other body organs. Megadoses of any one vitamin may inhibit the absorption of other nutrients.

At present, there is no reason to believe that large amounts of vitamins and minerals in supplement form will help to prevent or treat health problems or retard ageing processes.

Vitamin Supplements

Doctors occasionally prescribe dietary supplements to correct nutrient deficiencies. For example, dieters, heavy drinkers and those recovering from surgery or an illness may need certain supplements. Trauma and surgery increase the need for vitamin C for collagen synthesis. Some older people may not get the vitamins and minerals they need from their daily diet because of difficulty in getting or preparing their daily food.

Digestive problems, chewing difficulties and the use of certain drugs also interfere with good nutrition. People with these problems may benefit from a dietary supplement. If you are taking diuretics, you may require extra potassium. Check with your doctor about which supplements you should take.

Calcium and Vitamin D

Older people should pay particular attention to their need for calcium. Osteoporosis, or 'brittle bones', is preventable. A diet rich in calcium and vitamin D and a lifestyle that includes regular weight-bearing exercises are the best ways to prevent osteoporosis. The recommended total daily calcium intake for all Singaporean adults above age 19 is 700 mg. Calcium is found in several sources, but if necessary the recommended calcium intake may be fulfilled with calcium supplements.

Healthy foods rich in calcium are:

- low-fat dairy products such as cheese, yogurt and milk
- canned fish with edible bones like sardines and salmon
- dark green leafy vegetables such as *kai lan* or broccoli
- legumes such as beans and peas
- bread made with calcium-fortified flour.

Your body needs vitamin D to absorb calcium. The Osteoporosis Society (Singapore) recommends 400 IU of vitamin D daily for people below age 65, and 800 IU for those above 65. Being out in the sun for 15 minutes every day gives most people enough vitamin D. You also get this vitamin from supplements, as well as from cereals and milk fortified with vitamin D.

A Basic Diet Plan

Nutritionists have identified five food groups.

1. The bulk of a person's calorie requirements should come from grains (about 6–11 servings daily), a major source of complex carbohydrates, fibre and other nutrients. They may be taken in the form of rice and wheat flour and their products,

including bread, noodles and cereals. A serving amounts to a slice of bread, a cup of cooked rice or pasta or an ounce of dry cereal.

2. Vegetables are excellent sources of fibre, complex carbohydrates and essential vitamins and minerals. Take three to five servings daily. A serving of vegetables comprises one cup of leafy greens or half a cup of cooked carrots.

3. Eat two to four servings of fruit daily. Fruits provide fibre, natural sugars and complex carbohydrates. A serving of fruit comprises a medium-sized apple, pear or orange, a cup of diced fruit or a cup of fruit juice.

4. You should take two to three servings of dairy products daily. A serving of dairy products comprises one cup of milk or yogurt, or one-and-a-half ounces of cheese.

5. Eat two to three small servings of meat, poultry, fish, dried beans and peas, nuts and eggs daily. They are rich in protein, calcium and minerals. The total daily servings should add up to six ounces. Fish is a good source of protein.

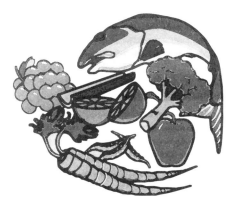

Ingredients for a basic diet plan

Getting the Most Out of Vegetables and Fruit

Vegetables and fruit provide the fibre and vitamins needed. Although you may be getting the correct quantity in the raw ingredients, the storage and preparation of these foods can change their essential value.

Choose the best. Not all foods are created equal. As a general principle, the darker the food, the more nutrients it contains. Pink grapefruit contains 30 times the vitamin A than the white variety. Some nutrient-packed vegetables are broccoli, spinach, peas, asparagus, sweet potatoes, carrots and red capsicum.

Eat fresh fruit and vegetables as soon as possible.
They lose half their vitamin C after two or three days in the refrigerator, and even faster at room temperature. If you cannot buy them fresh, buy them frozen. Freezing retains most of the nutrients.

Store food correctly. Heat, light and exposure to air or water destroy certain nutrients. Do not cut or wash fruit and vegetables before storing them. Do not soak or leave them in water. Water-soluble vitamins dissolve into the cooking water. The more water used, the more vitamins are wasted.

Minimise cutting. Chopping exposes the cut surfaces to air, causing oxidation of certain nutrients, especially vitamins A, C, B_6, thiamine and biotin. Cut in big chunks to minimise nutrient loss. Wait until the last minute before chopping or thawing.

Eat the whole thing. The outer layer of a plant is usually where most of the nutrients are concentrated. The outer green leaves of a cabbage contain more calcium, iron and vitamin A than the pale inner leaves. Scrub instead of peeling carrots and potatoes. The skin also prevents vitamin loss during cooking.

Choose good cooking methods. In general, fast cooking at relatively high temperatures is the best method. Therefore, stir-frying is the best method for retaining nutrients, followed by pressure-cooking and steaming. Boiling and deep-frying are the worst.

More Healthy Food Tips

1. Fats and sugars should be eaten sparingly.

2. Eat less processed foods. They have more calories and fewer nutrients than fresh foods.

3. If you enjoy snacking between meals, eat nourishing snacks. Most snacks add extra calories or salt to your diet, and have few vitamins and minerals. So, instead of candy, cake, cookies, potato chips, pretzels, take fruit, vegetable sticks, nuts, yogurt, cheese and crackers, bread and cereals.

4. Water is often dubbed the forgotten nutrient. Older people do not have a strong thirst sensation. Particularly when exercising in Singapore's hot weather, you will need to replace the water that you lose through perspiration. Taking highly salted food and caffeinated beverages will increase your body's water requirement.

Other Factors that Can Influence Food Intake and the Nutrition of the Older Person

1. Loss of teeth reduces chewing ability. This affects food choices and may lead to decreased intake of fruit, vegetables and meat, which are important sources of dietary fibre and protein. The ability to chew with dentures is significantly reduced compared to chewing with natural teeth. Dentures may also change the texture and taste of food. Dentures that do not fit well will cause discomfort, and make eating a burden rather than a joy.

2. Difficulty in swallowing is not normal. Consult a doctor to find out the cause, as the choice of treatment will depend on it. The problem may be neurological, such as the result of a stroke or Parkinson's Disease. If so, drugs and training in swallowing, in addition to adjusting the food consistency, can ease swallowing sufficiently to maintain adequate nutrition. If the problem is an obstruction that causes food to be stuck

in the throat, for instance a tumour or scarring from previous injury, surgery may be required. See 'Alternatives to Oral Feeding' opposite.

3. Social isolation

4. Financially dependent older people often opt for less expensive food which may be less nutritious or have a higher salt content (e.g., canned or preserved foods). Other expenditure (rent, medication) also compete with money spent on food, as illustrated in Madam Lee's case.

5. People with depression or dementia may have poor appetite, lose feelings of hunger, or feel no joy in eating.

6. Elders who find it difficult to walk or stand may be unable to prepare meals. Some have difficulty feeding themselves.

7. Alcohol gives calories without the nutritious content and may contribute to obesity.

8. Cigarettes may compete for money spent on food, while smoking alters taste sensations, usually making food less palatable, and eating becomes less enjoyable as a result.

The Dilemma of Mr S.S. and his Wife

Mr S.S. began having early symptoms of Parkinson's Disease at age 64. Over the years, his symptoms worsened. At age 73, his wife noticed that he took more than two hours to finish a meal. When he drank water, he would cough or water would spurt from his nose.

One night, he had difficulty breathing. He had a lot of phlegm at the back of his throat and started to run a fever. He was admitted to a geriatric ward with a diagnosis of aspiration pneumonia, a chest infection caused by foreign particles such as food going into the windpipe and lungs instead of the gullet and stomach. While a course of antibiotics was started for the pneumonia, a swallowing assessment revealed that it was unsafe for him to take food orally. In addition, he could not get enough daily nutrition orally because of the excessively long time he would take to finish a small portion of food.

Alternatives to Oral Feeding

If a person is not eating enough or is unable to swallow, alternatives to oral feeding may be required. Enteral nutrition involves putting food via a tube into the stomach or upper intestines. Home tube feeding can be a safe and effective therapy for many elders in need of nutritional support.

When enteral nutrition of less than three to six months is anticipated, tube feeding is usually done by inserting a small bore tube (naso-gastric tube) through a nostril and passing it into the stomach. When it is clear that tube feeding is going to be permanent, or if the disease is progressive, the doctor may suggest the patient be fed via a tube that leads directly into the stomach or small intestine. Siting the tube requires a minor surgical procedure called a percutaneous endoscopic gastrostomy or PEG.

The Two Methods of Tube Feeding

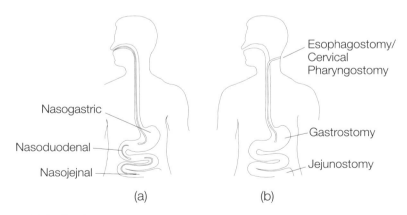

Tube feeding is done either through the nostril (a) or the stomach (b).

85

Choosing the Right Enteral Food

A patient on tube feeding will require liquid feeds. Such feeds can be 'total' or 'supplemental'. Supplemental feeding is carried out when a patient needs a nutrient preparation that is easy to prepare and take, to supplement an inadequate intake of food. Total enteral nutrition is usually prescribed for patients who cannot eat or drink because of unconsciousness, intestinal obstruction, certain diseases of the gut or the inability to swallow, from having a neurological disease.

Those who are alert and able to smell and taste home-made foods may blend home-cooked food for tube feeding. When preparing blended food, care must be taken to ensure adequate blending to prevent obstruction, cleanliness in preparation, and immediate refrigeration of unused portions to prevent bacterial contamination and growth. Commercial formulas have become popular because of their assured nutrient content, ease of preparation and sanitary packaging. Present-day enteral formulas have reached a high level of sophistication. They are manufactured from a variety of foods and chemicals to meet the different nutrient needs of patients.

There is a wide range of enteral preparations in the market. Standard preparations like Ensure,® Isocal,® Resource Standard®

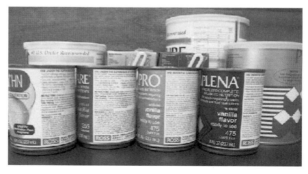

Supplementary feeds abound. Consult your doctor before buying any.

86

and Enercal® contain carbohydrates, proteins and fats in forms that require digestion and are designed to meet average nutritional needs. There are also many specialised enteral formulas, for example, Glucerna® and Resource Diabetic® for persons with diabetes mellitus, and Suplena® and Resource Renal® for those with kidney diseases.

Specialised products may be prescribed by a doctor in consultation with a registered dietitian. Consult your doctor on the appropriate choice of enteral formula. The Alexandra Geriatric Centre has prepared a patient education brochure on tube feeding.

8

Getting To The Root Of Pain

A Necessary Evil

Pain is defined by the Oxford dictionary as 'bodily suffering caused by injury or disease'. The medical concept of pain is that of a noxious (unpleasant) sensory and emotional experience associated with actual or potential tissue damage. Pain is subjective and varies between individuals who have different thresholds for it.

It is one of the most ubiquitous symptoms in daily life and is experienced by every human being at some time or other: babies, young adults and the elderly. In fact about 25 per cent of those above 65 years of age have problems with persistent pain and the incidence is higher in those who are debilitated. A local study found that 49 per cent of institutionalised elderly patients have some form of arthritic pain.

"Pain is a necessary evil," goes the saying. A famous theologian observed that pain was necessary for humans to survive in this world. Looking at lepers, one would appreciate the truth in this observation. Leprosy is a disease caused by an organism that affects the peripheral nerves supplying the extremities. It results in loss of sensation or numbness. Consequently, the involved extremities are subjected to repeated trauma without the sufferer being aware of it. This can lead to serious consequences such as ulcers, gangrene and even loss of limbs.

Pain, in a certain sense, acts as an indicator that something is amiss in the functioning of the bodily systems.

It is important to note that pain has multidimensional facets. Pain affects the person as a whole — not only physically but psychologically, emotionally and socially as well. A person suffering prolonged or repetitive severe pain experiences physical changes (racing pulse rate, sweating), psychological reactions (anxiety, fear, nervousness, insomnia, restlessness) and emotional reactions (sadness, self-pity). There are also social consequences including isolation, inability to take part in pleasurable pursuits and avoidance by others.

On the other hand, emotional, psychological and social factors are known to modulate the experience of pain and how one reacts and copes with it. For example, a person who is depressed or lonely tends to feel more pain than a person who is happy or has lots of social interaction with others, even if the pain is of similar intensity.

Let me share with you a few true cases to illustrate some common pain syndromes that can occur in the elderly.

Chest Pain

Mr Tan, a 68-year-old man, used to work as a building contractor. He had smoked heavily since the age of 20. He had been seeing me regularly at my clinic for control of high blood pressure and diabetes. He was noted to be well on most of his visits.

One day, while climbing a flight of stairs to his flat on the second level, he suddenly felt a sharp pain in the centre of his chest. It was excruciating, almost 'crushing' in nature, and sweat was pouring profusely over his forehead, neck and palms. He felt faint and nearly passed out. This forced him to rest on the floor in front of his flat. The pain persisted, but to a lesser degree. When the children came back, they helped him into the house and the pain soon subsided.

Later that day, I received a call from Mr Tan, who asked to bring forward his appointment with me. But upon hearing his complaint, I advised him to go to the emergency department at the hospital where I have a clinic. His symptoms certainly were worrying, although he tried to play them down and attributed it all to 'muscle pull' while climbing stairs. Just as I had suspected, he had suffered a heart attack, or in medical jargon, a myocardial infarct. He was subsequently admitted to the coronary care unit.

The way the above case unfolds is almost a classical study for a heart attack. The onset of the pain is usually sudden. It may be associated with exertion and has been variously described as 'constricting', 'crushing', or 'a vague tightness in the chest'.

People who have experienced a heart attack have described it as a frightening experience where they felt as if they were going to die. It is a 'feeling of doom'. The pain from the central region of the chest may project to the neck, jaw or shoulder tip. Cold sweat that comes with any chest pain should always be taken seriously as this has sinister implications. Other symptoms that may be associated with a heart attack are palpitations (sensation of a pounding heart), breathlessness and syncope (a fainting spell).

Less severe cardiac chest pain that comes on intermittently as a result of exertion and which is relieved by rest is known as angina pectoris. For a person with an underlying heart problem who experiences such attacks, the first step is to take a rest by sitting or lying down immediately and to place a tablet of glyceryl trinitrate (GTN) under the tongue. The tablet will dissolve and be absorbed from the mouth. The tablets are rendered less effective if swallowed instead of being absorbed from the mouth. Should angina persist after taking two to three tablets of sublingual (under the tongue) GTN, a heart attack may be imminent and the best course of action is to visit the doctor or go straight to the emergency department.

There are many other kinds of chest pain, but most are not quite like that caused by a heart attack. Nevertheless, it would be important to note some other causes of chest pain.

Chest pain can be musculoskeletal, meaning that it is caused by the muscles of the chest wall or skeletal structures: ribs, sternum, shoulder blades and collar bones. This is arguably the commonest cause of chest pain. One is able to identify this kind of pain by its mechanical nature; the pain, usually a dull ache, is triggered or exacerbated by movement or mechanical pressure.

Another type of chest pain that can be mistaken for a heart attack is oesophageal pain. This is usually due to reflux of the gastric juices into the lower oesophagus, causing an inflammation (also called oesophagitis). This pain has been described as heartburn or a burning sensation in the lower chest or upper abdomen. The pain is usually brought on by lying flat or by physical exertion, especially soon after a meal.

Chest pain that is brought on by deep breathing or cough may have a musculoskeletal cause. If associated with fever, cough or breathlessness, it could be due to inflammation of the membrane enveloping the thoracic cavity (pleuritis). The latter is usually associated with pneumonia or infection of the lung tissue. Occasionally, it can be due to a malignancy (tumour) of the lung.

Other less common but more serious causes of chest pain include aortic dissection and pulmonary embolism. The former refers to the splitting of the thoracic or abdominal aortic wall by a column of blood. The pain is usually very severe, described as sharp, shearing or tearing, and is usually projected to the back, between the shoulder blades or the limbs. Most people who suffer this have long-standing hypertension.

Pulmonary embolism, on the other hand, is usually due to a blood clot in a vein that has migrated from the legs, pelvis or lower abdomen to a pulmonary artery. This causes obstruction and the cessation of blood supply to a section of the lung. Persons at especially high risk of pulmonary embolism are those with blood clots in the deep veins of the legs (deep vein thrombosis). They include those who are obese and immobile as a result of a stroke or lower limb fracture.

Joint Pain

Seventy-year-old Madam Lim had been a housewife all her life. She was overweight, had a long history of diabetes and hypertension, and was on follow-up visits to her general practitioner. She had been keeping well, except for a nagging pain in her knees. This pain had worsened over the past four to five years.

The pain, which was described as dull and aching, worsened as the day wore on. It was especially painful after walking or standing for prolonged periods and was relieved after a rest. It could last from days to weeks. Madam Lim also noticed that on certain occasions the pain was associated with swelling and tenderness of both her knee joints. Lately, the knees had also begun to feel a little stiff, and there was a grating sensation whenever she flexed them.

It was only after the knee problems started interfering with her daily activities that she decided to seek further treatment. When she saw me during the consultation, I noticed that she was walking with a limp, grimacing in pain with every step she took. Her knees were deformed and swollen, and when the knee joint was moved, I could feel a sensation of 'roughness' (or crepitus). A diagnosis of osteoarthritis of the knees was made and this was confirmed with X-rays of the knees.

Osteoarthritis of the knee is a fairly common condition in the elderly. It is a degenerative condition where, as a result of wear and tear, the cartilage covering the ends of the bones (femur and tibia) that make up the knee joint lose their elasticity. As a result there is pain, swelling and stiffness of the knees. This pain becomes worse after a period of sustained use of the knees.

Musculoskeletal ailments of the muscles, joints or bones are quite common in the elderly. Musculoskeletal pain, as alluded to earlier, is usually brought on by mechanical pressure and movement, and the pain may cease once these precipitating causes are removed. The pain can range from a dull ache to the excruciating pain experienced in a fractured bone.

Other common musculoskeletal pain syndromes in the elderly can occur in the shoulders and back. The 'painful arc syndrome' which is also known as frozen shoulder refers to a painful condition of the shoulder where the affected person experiences pain on trying to lift his or her arm.

The pain may occur within a certain range of movement (hence the term 'painful arc') or may be so severe that the affected person is unable to lift the arm at all ('frozen' arm). This condition is also due to wear and tear, which results in inflammation of the tendons forming the shoulder joint capsule.

Back pain is a frequent complaint among the elderly. This can occur spontaneously or after an injury to the back. Spontaneous back pain can also result from degenerative changes in the joints of the spine (the facet joints and the intervertebral joints and discs). This is termed spondylosis and may involve the lumbar or thoracic spine or both together.

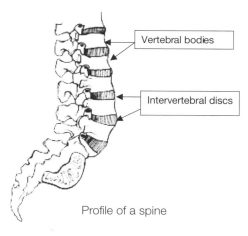

Profile of a spine

One of the most common back pains is that which occurs after a fall where one lands on one's buttocks. In the elderly, the spine may be osteoporotic (having reduced bone mass) and even minor trauma can lead to compression fractures of the vertebral bodies of the spine. The resulting back pain is exacerbated by movement. In fact it may be so bad that the affected person is unable to stand up, let alone walk. This in turn curtails the person's mobility and impairs his or her daily activities.

Another fracture that occurs frequently in those with osteoporotic bones is fracture of the hip bones. The pain is localised in the hip joint, that is, around the upper thigh, groin or buttock region. The person is unable to stand up, and the affected leg is rotated outwards and appears shortened. In most cases, admission to hospital is recommended.

In general, musculoskeletal or joint pain can be treated with oral painkillers, or analgesics. A common painkiller is paracetamol (e.g., Panadol), which raises the pain threshold. It does this by inhibiting the formation and action of chemicals mediating pain, and acts at the nerve pathways that convey the pain sensation. Other painkillers include synthetic forms of opiates like morphine, tramadol (e.g., Tramal®), buprenorphine (e.g., Temgesic®) and codeine. Some analgesics like Panadeine are derived from a combination of both paracetamol and codeine. Painkillers that act by reducing inflammation are usually referred to as Non-Steroid Anti-Inflammatory Drugs (NSAIDs). Examples of these are aspirin, mefenamic acid (Ponstan®), indomethacin (Indocid®), diclofenac sodium (Voltaren®), ketoprofen (Oruvail®) and naproxen (Naprosyn®).

Overconsumption of paracetamol may cause liver damage, while opiate derivatives may cause sedation, nausea, vomiting and giddiness. NSAIDs can cause peptic ulcers, gastritis, and in severe cases, even bleeding from the gut or kidney damage. These drugs should therefore be used with caution.

Measures for pain relief other than oral painkillers include physiotherapy, injection of steroids into the joint (alone or with anaesthetic agents), local heat treatment (ultraviolet or short-wave, warm towel, or a hotwater bag wrapped in a towel to prevent burning the skin), and applying topical painkiller gels such as ketoprofen, piroxicam gel, deep heat. Any painful joint should be rested, and the stress or weight transmitted through the affected joint should be reduced. This can be achieved by using a walking stick or frame.

Nerve Pain

Mr Chua had suffered from diabetes for more than 20 years. He was initially on oral medication but due to its ineffectiveness in controlling sugar levels, the medication was switched to insulin injections about five years prior to our meeting. Over the years he had developed multiple complications of diabetes. He required laser treatment for his eyes to prevent him from going blind, while his right big toe had been amputated because of an infected ulcer and gangrene.

In the past month or so before he came to see me at the clinic, he had started experiencing a painful sensation in his feet. He later described it as a feeling somewhere between 'a burning sensation' and 'stepping on pins and needles'. The pain progressed to the point where it affected his sleep badly. He had seen many GPs but to no avail. As a result he became depressed and irritable. Before long, his appetite was affected and his general condition deteriorated.

The pain that Mr Chua experienced is typical of 'nerve' or neuropathic pain. Pain can arise anywhere along the nervous system, from the peripheral nerves of the limbs to the spinal cord and finally to the brain itself. The nature of the pain has been variously described as a burning sensation, a sensation of 'pins and needles' or a sharp shooting pain almost like electric currents running down the affected limb. The pain described by Mr Chua is consistent with diabetic neuropathy. This usually occurs in patients with poorly controlled diabetes, where the nerves of the extremities are affected.

Treatment of this type of pain is often unsatisfactory. The various modes of treatment include:

- achieving a better control of blood glucose
- using simple analgesics like paracetamol
- using antidepressants like amitriptyline, imipramine, nor-triptyline
- 'stabilising' the nerves with high-dose vitamins (such as B complex, Neurobion® Methylcobal®) or anti-epileptic agents like carbamazepine (Tegretol®).
- applying Capsaicin topically as a cream may also be helpful for painful diabetic neuropathy.

Another type of neuropathic pain has a 'shooting' or sharp quality. This is usually experienced by an individual with a pro-lapsed intervertebral disc, the disc which separates one vertebral body from another. When the disc protrudes, it may impinge upon the nerve roots, thus causing pain. Most often, it is the lumbar spine that is involved.

Typically, the pain shoots down to the buttocks or down the side of the affected leg. The pain is exacerbated or precipitated by the straight leg-raising test, which requires the patient to raise the leg while keeping the knees straight. This stipulation ensures that the main movement is at the hips.

Quite often, neuropathic pain is associated with numbness or diminished sensation of the affected nerve or nerves. In severe and long-standing cases, this may result in weakness of the muscles supplied by the nerves. Treatment of this type of pain may include bed rest, traction (attaching weights to the painful leg) and simple painkillers. Occasionally, surgery by an orthopae-dic surgeon to remove the protruding disc(s) may be needed.

Colic Pain

Seventy-eight-year-old Madam Tan had been having problems with her bowel movements for the past 10 years. She had depended on laxatives every three to four days to open her bowels, and occasionally needed a suppository.

She was seen at the accident and emergency department of the hospital for severe abdominal pain, which she described as a twisting or squeezing pain in the lower abdomen which 'comes and goes' over minutes. The pain came on rather gradually, slowly built up to a peak, and then abated gradually. This occurred repeatedly and caused Madam Tan much distress. Incidentally, she had not emptied her bowels for 10 days prior to her hospital visit. Subsequent investigation in the hospital revealed that she had severe constipation colic.

Colic is characterised by a wrenching pain that waxes and wanes with time. It usually results from the propulsive and contractile action of a tubular structure in the body against an obstruction. The commonly affected tubular structures are the gastrointestinal tract (intestines), ureter (tube joining the kidneys to the bladder) and biliary tract (tube draining bile from the gall bladder and liver to the small intestine). The cause of the obstruction is usually the presence of a stone (especially in ureters or biliary tracts), stools (in the gut) or a tumour (possible in all three areas).

Colicky abdominal pain originating from the gut is very common. Even normal individuals experience it just before emptying their bowels or when they have diarrhoea. However, colicky pain with abdominal distension can be a sign of obstruction of the gut. This could be due to impacted stools, a tumour or a large gallstone. In the elderly, constipation is a common cause and is easily treatable.

Ureteric colic usually occurs when a stone from the kidney is being passed via the ureter to the urinary bladder. As the stone is being propelled downwards, a colicky pain is felt in the loin. This pain may radiate (project) towards the groin ('loin de groin' pain). The pain may be so intense that it may cause the victim to double up or even roll over in bed. This condition may be associated with bloodstained urine.

A stone that is being passed down the biliary tract, usually the common bile duct, causes colicky pain in the right upper abdominal region, just below the right rib cage. This may be associated with jaundice (yellow pigmentation of the skin and eyes) and infection of the tract because of stagnant bile.

The treatment of colicky pain should be determined by its cause. If the pain is due to constipation colic, treatment should be directed towards clearing the bowels. This can be done with a bowel washout, an enema, suppositories or oral laxatives (e.g., Lactulose, Bisacodyl, Senna). Pain from biliary colic may be relieved with an antispasmodic drug like hyoscine butylbromide (Buscopan®) or probantheline bromide (Pro-Banthine®). Antispasmodic drugs relieve pain by relaxing muscle contractions of the ureter or bile duct. If the pain is very severe, an opiate painkiller like pethidine may also be given. Surgery to remove the obstruction may be required.

The case examples given in this chapter describe briefly the types of pain commonly experienced by older persons. This list is, however, not exhaustive. There are many other types of pain that occur in different settings and it may be very difficult to pinpoint the exact cause even after numerous investigations in hospital. Pain that is persistent and that interferes with a person's daily activities or lifestyle should be subjected to a proper assessment by a doctor.

Pain is a common symptom in the elderly, but it is a necessary phenomenon because it alerts the body to the possibility of some abnormal process taking place, whether physical, psychological or emotional. Chronic pain is a multidimensional symptom that affects the whole person and conversely is affected by many factors both internal and external to the sufferer. Hence its treatment has to be multifaceted or multi-disciplinary in nature.

Apart from the physical aspect, the psychosocial, emotional and spiritual aspects of pain have also to be tackled. Prescribing potent painkillers may not suffice if the sufferer is depressed and socially isolated. Likewise, a person who uses pain as a way to gain attention and care from his loved ones (pain behaviour) would be none the better even with the strongest of analgesics. Pain has to be approached holistically.

We should therefore not underestimate the effects of alternative approaches to pain control. Among those that have been used are cognitive behavioural therapy, music therapy, art therapy, aromatherapy, acupuncture, meditation and relaxation therapy.

Pain in a person should not be allowed to persist for too long as it affects the whole person and those around him. Not only does it cause physical distress, psychological and emotional upheaval is experienced as well, while the social costs may also be significant. It is important, therefore, that the underlying cause of pain should be identified and tackled as quickly as possible.

9

When A Pill Is Not A Cure

A Pill for Every Ill?

Madam Tan, who is 70, had been having arthritis in both knees for five years. It started with pain in the knees while she was squatting or climbing stairs. Two years ago, she could not tolerate the 20-minute walk to the market and had to stop several times during each trip. She decided to see her family doctor, who gave her some 'anti-rheumatism' tablets to be taken daily. This proved to be of some help because it relieved her pain somewhat. However, she decided to cut down on her social activities in case her knees gave her more problems.

Over the next two years, she put on 10 kg. (At our first consultation she weighed 75 kg despite being only 1.5 metres tall.) Then her husband passed away after an illness, and she began to feel very lonely, especially as her daughter had married and moved out three years before. When her daughter invited her to stay with her for a few months, she accepted the invitation.

The daughter was concerned because her mother looked more lethargic than before, had problems sleeping at night, and her feet became swollen in the afternoons. That was when she found out that one doctor had given her mother vitamins to improve her 'energy', another had prescribed sleeping tablets to help her sleep, and a third had given 'water' tablets to reduce the swelling of her feet.

Madam Tan, in searching for a cure for all her woes, had been visiting any and every doctor in her neighbourhood — and probably beyond, too! After every visit, she would put all her tablets into one container so that it would be easier to find them. She thought she could remember them by their shape, colour and size. However, when the time came for her to take the medications, she became confused. All of them looked alike, and she had to go by her memory and 'impression' of the tablets to decide which ones to take. There were periods when she passed urine several times at night and felt very sleepy during the day. She was finally referred to me when she visited the polyclinic. I was probably the fifth or sixth doctor she had consulted over the past year!

A Confusing Consultation

Having heard the history of her complaints, I asked Madam Tan why she had consulted so many doctors. Her answer was typical of many of my patients:

"This is because Dr A is good for treating knee pain, and I was recommended to see Dr B because he is good for treating sleep problems, while Dr C is good for …"

Somehow, doctors are categorised as being good in treating one or two conditions only!

"So, can you tell me what medicine you are taking now?" I asked.

After a long pause she put her hand into her big bag and took out an equally big plastic bag bulging with medicine bottles. I thought I would have an easy time sorting through the various drugs, until I found that some had no labels on them, while others had been transferred to another bottle.

The labels and the tablets didn't match. All I saw were lots of tablets and capsules, many of which looked alike. She was equally baffled.

After going through the scraps of information that she could provide, and making numerous phone calls to the doctors she had consulted previously, I was finally able to piece together her problems. She was on a total of eight different types of medication, some had been duplicated because they were known by different trade names, and she was also mixed up about when the tablets were to be taken. She had 'medication-induced' disease!

'Medication-induced' Disease

'Medication-induced' disease is a condition whereby much of the person's illnesses and complaints are caused by the interaction and side effects of multiple drugs. Madam Tan had been prescribed a nonsteroidal, anti-inflammatory agent (NSAID) to relieve the pain in her arthritic knees. To counteract the effect of the NSAID on the stomach (as it could cause gastritis), she was given antacids as well. However, both NSAID and antacids are known to cause diarrhoea. When she contracted diarrhoea, she saw another doctor for it but did not inform him of the drugs she was taking for her arthritis. This doctor gave her a prescription of a constipating drug to stop the diarrhoea.

When she decided to cut down on her social activities to reduce further strain on her knees, this caused her to put on weight, which further stressed her arthritic knees. When this happened, the knee pain got worse, and heralded the prescription of even more painkillers. By the time I checked her medication, I found that she was taking a double dose of NSAID. Both were given by different doctors who did not know what other drugs she had been given. Neither did she.

When she went back home and compared the names, they were spelt differently and she assumed that they were different drugs. Such confusion may be caused when one clinic labels its medicine using trade names while another uses the generic name.

Examples are Ponstan (trade name) and mefenamic acid (generic name), Temgesic (trade name) and buprenorphine (generic name), Oruvail (trade name) and ketoprofen (generic name).

With her husband's death and her daughter's marriage, Madam Tan was left all alone at home. This sudden loneliness and her inability to go out of the house depressed her. She kept lying in bed thinking how fearful it was to 'die alone without anyone knowing'. The depression kept her awake at night. However, when faced with the doctor, she put on a brave front and just complained that she could not sleep. This led to a prescription of sleeping pills.

When her feet were swollen, a prescription of 'water' tablets was given. However, this swelling was absent in the morning and came on only in the evening. Moreover, she was not breathless when walking and she could lie flat in bed. A feeling of breathlessness upon lying flat in bed (or orthopnoea) may be suggestive of accumulation of water in the lungs, and could indicate heart failure. The swelling of her legs was the result of gravity and the NSAID that she was taking. NSAID is known to cause salt and water retention.

And of course, Madam Tan had mixed up the water tablets and sleeping pills. By taking the water tablets at night, she passed urine frequently in the night, thus disturbing her sleep. By taking the sleeping tablets in the morning, she became very sleepy in the day.

How to Prevent 'Medication-induced' Disease

It is not difficult to prevent 'medication-induced' disease. However, it does require some effort. Here are some guidelines:

1. Inform your doctor of any drug allergies. When you are told that you have a drug allergy, find out the name of the medicine. It is not enough to know that you have an allergy without knowing what you are allergic to. If possible, ask your

doctor to apply for a 'Medic Awas' card for you. This card documents your drug allergies and includes the name of the doctor who made the diagnosis (in case a counter-check is needed later on).

2. Relate your entire medical history to your doctor. The presence of certain medical conditions precludes the use of certain types of medication. For example, the presence of asthma precludes the use of propranolol and related drugs for the treatment of high blood pressure; and the presence of gastric problems, and especially a history of bleeding gastric ulcers, precludes the use of anti-inflammatory agents like NSAIDs.

3. Take all your medications along when you see the doctor. This will help to avoid duplication of the same drugs. It will also help the doctor to stop unnecessary medication.

4. Leave the labels on medicine containers. Do not rely on your memory as it may fail you at the crucial moment. Do not rely on the shape and colour because they may change with different 'batches' or with different drug companies.

5. If you have difficulty remembering when to take the various medications, use a pillbox, and ask your family to pack them for you. A pillbox usually has four separate compartments. You can label them with the time of day or mark them with symbols. For example, use the symbol of a rising sun for drugs to be taken in the morning, full sun for those to be taken at noon, and the moon for night doses. All the medicine that is to be taken at one particular time can be packed into a compartment. An alarm clock or phone call from someone in the family can help to prompt forgetful persons to take their medicine.

6. Tell the doctor if you are confused over your medication. Your doctor may be able to simplify the medication list. It can be extremely frustrating to conform to a complex dosing regime, such as: "Take half of tablet A and one of tablet B

before meals, two tablets of C after your morning meal, one tablet of B and one tablet of D in the afternoon, half a table-spoon of E at 5.00 pm, one tablet of A, B and C after dinner, and one of tablet F before bedtime." As far as possible, ask for a simpler alternative.

7. Don't doctor-hop. Doctors are trained to look after every part of the body. A doctor can be effective only if he has all the information about you and your condition. The trouble with doctor-hopping is that each doctor would know only a part of your medical history. With limited information, it would be difficult to make an accurate diagnosis, without which no treatment would be possible. So, stick to one doctor you can relate with.

8. Don't pressurise your doctor into giving you medicine. I have come across many patients who would not leave my consultation room until they felt satisfied that they had received 'a pill for every ill'. It is not necessary that a tablet be prescribed for every minor complaint. For example, cough mixtures containing antihistamines will also stop your cough and running nose without the need for a separate prescription.

    Medicines are not a 'cure-all' and they do not turn back the clock. Some conditions are a result of old age while others are due to injuries sustained in one's youth. Learning to accept them as they are may stop many from doctor-hopping in search of the elusive cure.

9. Over-the-counter (OTC) medicines are forms of medication, too. So remember to tell your doctor which other medicines you are taking on your own. These include drugs like paracetamol, aspirin and even vitamins.

10. Do not rely excessively on medication. You may be able to reduce some forms of medication (on doctor's orders only) that you are taking with some common sense. For example, reducing your weight can decrease stress on a diseased joint

and so reduce the need for painkillers. You can reduce smokers' cough by quitting smoking instead of relying on cough mixtures. Appropriate dieting can lower blood pressure, improve diabetic or lipid control, and may in turn reduce the amount of drugs you need to take.

Medicine is a double-edged sword. When used correctly, it can relieve pain and suffering. When abused, it does more harm than good, and may in itself be the cause of many unpleasant symptoms it was meant to treat. Skilful prescribing is possible only when there is full knowledge about the patient's complaints, current prescribed medication and previous medical history. Both the doctor and the patient must share this responsibility.

As for Madam Tan, her last question to me was, "So doctor, what medicine are you going to give me now?" It took me a long time to convince (and educate) her to accept that what she needed was not more but less medicine. I suppose some habits are hard to change.

A Guide to Proper Medicine-taking

a) Do's

1. Follow instructions exactly — there are good reasons why some medications must be taken in a particular manner.

2. Swallow your medicine with sufficient water.

3. Let your doctor know if there are side effects.

4. Get to know your medicine.

5. Keep a daily record of the time medicine is taken in a book — this may prevent you from missing a dose or taking double doses of the same medicine by mistake.

6. Take all the medications that you are on, including OTC drugs, with you when you see your doctor.

b) Don'ts

1. Don't take different types of medication together — ask your doctor how and when to take them.

2. Don't assume that medicine given for a previous illness is suitable for your present problem.

3. Don't take medicine that is prescribed for other people — even if the symptoms are the same. The same medicine can have very different effects on another person.

4. Don't take your medicine in the dark — you may take the wrong one.

5. Don't lose or mix up the labels for your medicine — they may be alike in size, shape and colour.

10

Choosing The Right Senior Care Service

In recent times, there has been no lack of services and facilities for the older person. Sometimes, we end up not making use of any of these services because we do not know what they are for, and do not see the benefits they offer. It is true that making use of an unsuitable service or facility is of no help and could be worse than not making use of any at all.

Let me illustrate with a few examples how some services can be utilised 'skilfully' to help us look after the older ones at home and to improve our own wellbeing.

Day Care Centres

Madam Toh, 77, suffered a stroke, after which she could walk a few steps at a time with the aid of a walking frame but was too weak to go out of the house. She lived with her son and daughter-in-law, both of whom worked during the day. As she used to be active before her stroke, she became withdrawn, depressed and lonely during the long hours that she was left alone at home. Madam Toh's concerned son arranged for a consultation with me because she was losing weight and was often weepy.

During the consultation, I discovered that when she was left alone, she took to bed because time passed 'faster' when she was asleep. She started skipping lunch as 'it was no fun eating alone', day after day. As a result, she was losing weight and becoming malnourished.

As a doctor, I could treat her depression and perhaps even her weight loss with medication and the nutritional supplements that can be bought at the pharmacy. But there is no pill to treat loneliness. Hence, I referred her to a day care centre. It took much convincing before she and her family agreed to the suggestion. Somehow, some of them still think it is an old folks' home!

There are three types of day care centres: social day care centres, rehabilitative day centres and day hospitals for patients with dementia.

Social Day Care Centres

Social day care centres cater to the social needs of the older person and most have trained staff who can meet these needs. Programmes for the elderly can be quite structured. There are group activities (for mental and physical stimulation), updates of current affairs (beneficial for those who cannot read newspapers or watch news broadcasts), games, counselling sessions, educational talks on health and other social activities. These are interspersed with physical exercises.

The centres are equipped with simple devices for the older person to train with, such as exercise pedals, parallel bars, pulleys, and so on. Of course, the programmes differ from one centre to another. Meals and transport are usually provided. Clients may attend such centres from one to five days a week. Fees charged also vary among the different centres.

Rehabilitative Day Centres

These are similar in many respects to social day care centres, but there is emphasis on the 'exercise training' component. In these centres, you would expect to find a physiotherapist and/or an occupational therapist working with the elderly, individually or in a group. The range of equipment available is also wider and more sophisticated than in a social day care centre, and includes treadmill machines, heating devices and the like. This is an ideal setting for the older person who has recently suffered a disability and is expected to improve over time with rehabilitation. I have seen patients being admitted into such centres in a wheelchair, and later walking out the door on their own upon being discharged from the programme.

Day Hospitals

Offering an even higher level of intensive outpatient rehabilitation than rehabilitative day centres, day hospitals are usually situated within acute regional hospitals, and have the full medical team comprising the geriatrician, specially trained staff nurses, therapists and social workers. Clients attending such centres are frail and require more intensive therapy than those in rehabilitative day centres.

Madam Toh was referred to a centre with both social and rehabilitation components. She attended the rehabilitation day centre twice a week and the adjoining social day care centre the remaining three weekdays. This gave her an avenue for socialisation, so relieving her feelings of boredom and loneliness, and at the same time allowing her to work out those muscles which had been wasting away from underuse.

Such benefits were not just limited to Madam Toh. While she was at the centre, her son and daughter-in-law had peace of mind, knowing that she was safe and supervised, and they did not need to phone to check on her while they were at work. After a period of rehabilitation, she was strong enough to do a lot for herself, and this lessened the need for her family to assist her at home or on weekends.

Another type of day care centre is for patients with dementia. These centres function like social day care centres. The environment is altered to suit the needs of the clients, and the staff are trained in managing patients with dementia and its associated behavioural problems, like disorientation, mood changes or the tendency to wander.

If people suffering from moderate to severe dementia are placed in a social day care centre, it could be most disruptive to the centre and would not benefit such persons at all. Similarly, it would not benefit (and may even harm) a frail person in need of rehabilitation to be sent to a centre meant for those with dementia. Hence, the correct choice of day centre is important for both the patient and the family. This chapter ends with lists of the various care centres for the elderly.

Home Help Services and Befrienders' Services

What if Madam Toh and her family had adamantly refused day care? What else could have been done then? Well, we would have had to think of providing some kind of care for her at home.

Home help services are provided to help older persons who stay at home who would otherwise have difficulty performing household tasks for themselves. Hence, these services cater to older persons who are left alone at home for long durations. The services include meal delivery, laundry service, purchase of daily necessities, home management (like cleaning and tidying the house), personal hygiene (including bathing) and escort services (such as accompanying the older person to medical appointments). There is a minimal charge for providing such services and fees are levied based on the ability to pay.

The Befrienders' Service take on roles similar to those of home helpers. 'Befrienders' are usually groups of volunteers who become friends with the lonely elderly at home. Their visits help to reduce the boredom and loneliness such elders face.

Respite Care Services

Respite care is another misunderstood service. Caring for the older person is a very difficult task. It is not a '9 to 5' job, but often a 24-hour one; and it can be physically and emotionally draining for the caregiver. The children of some of my patients have not had a holiday for the past 10 years, ever since they began caring for their elderly parents at home.

Although many caregivers put on a brave front, I know they are, deep down, very tired and drained. When burnout occurs, the quality of care given to their loved ones diminishes. In extreme cases, burnout may even lead to anger, elder abuse and outright rejection. When this takes place, the problem can be emotionally challenging for the caregivers who face conflicting emotions of guilt and frustration.

Hence, I have always made it a point to advise the family on respite care. When the caregiver feels very tired and needs a break, he or she could arrange for the elderly loved one to be 'admitted' to a respite care facility, which could be a community hospital or a nursing home.

Once the elder is admitted, the family members can take a break from the caring, go on holiday or do something they had always wanted to do, but hitherto had not found the time to. After such a break, they often return more relaxed, emotionally recharged and ready to take on the caregiving role again. Caring will not be seen as such a burden because there is now an outlet for them in times of need. This option could be recommended for Madam Toh's family.

Domiciliary Care

When the older person becomes housebound and has no access to geriatric services, due perhaps to the lack of caregivers or to a severe disability, care must go to the person 'trapped' at home. This is known as a domiciliary service. It could involve one or a few of the following: home visits by a doctor (domiciliary medical service), home nursing or home therapy. These services are generally expensive. There are some voluntary organisations providing such services and they usually have strict criteria to prevent abuse.

Lists of the various homecare services available for the elderly can be found at the end of this chapter. The lists are not comprehensive. They are meant to indicate where some of these services are found.

A Caregiver's Homecare Guide

A. How to Change a Bedbound Patient's Bedsheet

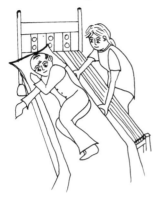

1. Turn the bedridden person to one side. Use a pillow to support the body. Roll up the soiled bedsheet.

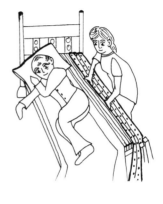

2. Put on a clean bedsheet, leaving enough material to tuck it in.

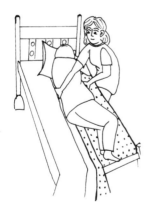

3. Turn and support the person with a pillow. Pull soiled bedsheet away.

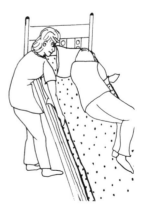

4. Remove the soiled bedsheet. Pull clean bedsheet so that it is wrinkle-free.

B. How to Give a Bedbath

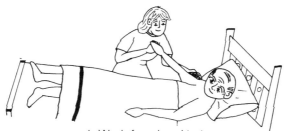

1. Wash from head to toe.

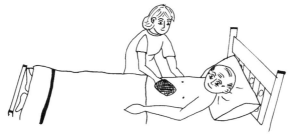

2. Move sheet and towel down to the waist. Expose only the area that is being cleaned.

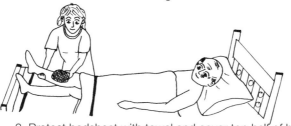

3. Protect bedsheet with towel and cover top half of body while washing the legs.

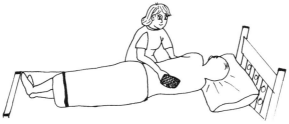

4. Turn the bedridden person to one side and clean the back.

C. How to Clean a Wound

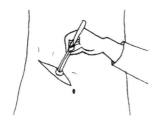

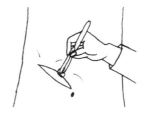

1. Begin by washing your hands. First swab the centre of the wound with clean cotton dipped in saline solution.

2. Next, clean the edges using another clean cotton swab.

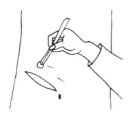

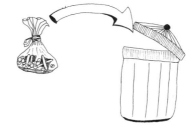

3. Finally, clean the areas surrounding the wound. Wash your hands before applying the dressing.

4. Put all used materials and soiled dressings in a plastic bag before disposal.

* Clean with normal saline unless otherwise indicated.

D. Areas prone to pressure sores must be carefully monitored. Barrier creams and turning at two-hour intervals are two preventive measures.

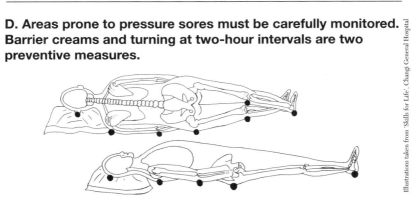

Illustrations taken from 'Skills for Life', Changi General Hospital

E. How to Use Walking Aids

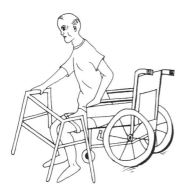

Chair to Walker Transfer

- Apply wheelchair brakes.
- The caregiver stands on the user's weaker or injured side.
- The user pushes on the armrests of the wheelchair to stand up.
- The user holds on to the frame with his stronger hand, then places the other hand on the frame.

Walking with a Walker

- The caregiver stands behind the user on his weaker or injured side.
- The user picks up the walker and stands behind it.
- The user should avoid sliding the walker, but always lift it as he moves forward.
- Check that all legs are on the floor.
- The user steps forward with the weaker leg/side and follows through with the other leg.

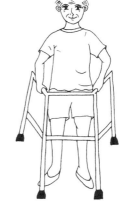

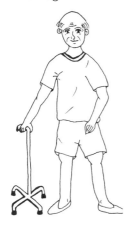

Walking with a Stick

- The caregiver stands on the same side as the user's weaker or injured leg.
- The user should hold the stick in the stronger hand.
- The user moves the weaker leg forward first, and follows with the stronger leg.

Illustrations taken from 'Skills for Life', Changi General Hospital

117

Some Social Day Care Centres

Apex Day Care for the Elderly
Blk 119 Bukit Merah View #01-85, Singapore 152119.
Tel: 2734510

Ayer Rajah Day Care Centre
300 Teban Gardens, Singapore 609342. Tel: 5623037

May Wong Social Centre for the Elderly
Blk 117 Bukit Merah View #01-205, Singapore 15211.
Tel: 2706654

Salvation Army Bedok Multi-Service Centre for the Elderly
Blk 121 Bedok North Road #01-16, Singapore 460121.
Tel: 4451630

Salvation Army Peacehaven Nursing Home for the Aged
9 Upper Changi Road North, Singapore 507706.
Tel: 5465678

The Wan Qing Lodge
Blk 236 #01-346 Jurong East St 21, Singapore 600236.
Tel: 5692131

Home Nursing Foundation Rehabilitative Day Care Centres

The Home Nursing Foundation (HNF) has a number of rehabilitative day care centres called Senior Citizens' Health Care Centres. They are:

Ang Mo Kio Senior Citizens' Health Care Centre
Ang Mo Kio Community Hospital (Level 2)
17 Ang Mo Kio Ave 9, Singapore 569766. Tel: 4506152

Bukit Batok Polyclinic
50 Bukit Batok West Ave 3, Singapore 659164. Tel: 5634476

Hougang Senior Citizens' Health Care Centre
Hougang Polyclinic (Level 3).
89 Hougang Ave 4, Singapore 538829. Tel: 3820274

Geylang Senior Citizens' Health Care Centre
Geylang Polyclinic (Level 4)
21 Geylang East Central, Singapore 389707. Tel: 7468671

Tampines Senior Citizens' Health Care Centre
Tampines Polyclinic (Level 3)
1 Tampines Street 41, Singapore 529203. Tel: 7865373

Toa Payoh Senior Citizens' Health Care Centre
Toa Payoh Polyclinic (Level 3)
2003 Toa Payoh Lor 8, Singapore 319260. Tel: 2590669

Other Rehabilitative Day Care Centres

Apex Rehabilitation Centre for the Elderly
Blk 119 #01-51, Singapore 152119. Tel: 2719685

Day Care Centre for the Elderly
Ling Kwang Home for Senior Citizens
156 Serangoon Garden Way, Singapore 556055. Tel: 2875466

METTA Day Rehabilitation Centre for the Elderly
Blk 296 Tampines St 22 #01-526, Singapore 520296.
Tel: 7895951

St Andrew's Community Hospital Day Rehabilitation Centre
1 Elliot Road, Singapore 458686. Tel: 2419956

Day Hospitals

Alexandra Geriatric Centre
Alexandra Hospital, 378 Alexandra Road, Singapore 59964.
Tel: 4708415

Geriatric Day Hospital
Changi General Hospital, 2 Simei St 3, Singapore 529889.
Tel: 8502969

Day Care Centres for Patients with Dementia

New Horizon Centre (Toa Payoh)
Blk 151 #01-468 Lor 2 Toa Payoh, Singapore 310151.
Tel: 3538734

New Horizon Centre (Bt Batok)
Blk 511 #01-211 Bt Batok St 52, Singapore 650511.
Tel: 5659958

Apex Harmony Lodge
10 Pasir Ris Walk (off Pasir Ris Drive), Singapore 518240.
Tel: 5852265

Thong Teck Home Day Care Centre
91 Geylang East Ave 2, Singapore 523941.
Tel: 8460069

Home Help Services

Dorcas Home Care Service
The Presbyterian Welfare Services
Blk 156A #01-01 Mei Chin Rd
Brickwork Town Council, Singapore 140150.
Tel: 4762630

Touch Community Services
3615 Jalan Bukit Merah, 3rd floor Touch Community Theatre,
Singapore 159461.
Tel: 3770122

Respite Care Facilities

St Andrew's Community Hospital
1 Elliot Road, Singapore 458686.
Tel: 2419956

St Luke's Hospital for the Elderly
2 Bukit Batok St 11, Singapore 659674.
Tel: 5632281

Ang Mo Kio Community Hospital
17 Ang Mo Kio Ave 9, Singapore 569766.
Tel: 4541729

Kwong Wai Shiu Hospital
705 Serangoon Road, Singapore 328127.
Tel: 2993747/ 2945637

Befrienders' Services

Ang Mo Kio Social Service Centre
Blk 230 #01-1264 Ang Mo Kio Ave 3, Singapore 560230.
Tel: 4535349

Bukit Ho Swee Social Service Centre
Blk 26 #01-42/52 Jalan Klinik, Singapore 160026. Tel: 2742646

Kang Ning Centre for the Elderly
Blk 228 #01-45 Bt Batok Central, Singapore 650228.
Tel: 5690579

Geylang East Home for the Aged
Blk 97 #01-439 Aljunied Crescent, Singapore 380097.
Tel: 7457880

Telok Ayer Hong Lim Green Community Centre Senior Citizens Club
Blk 533 Upper Cross Street #05-214
Hong Lim Complex, Singapore 050533. Tel: 5344002

Islamic Religious Council (Majlis Ugama Islam Singapura)
273 Braddell Road, Singapore 579702. Tel: 2568188

Lions Befriender Service Association
Blk 130 #01-358 Bukit Merah View, Singapore 150130.
Tel: 3758600

MacPherson Moral Family Service Centre
Blk 91 #01-3023 Paya Lebar Way, Singapore 370091.
Tel: 7414255

Muslim Missionary Society Singapore (JAMIYAH)
31 Lorong 12 Geylang, Singapore 399006. Tel: 7431211

PERTAPIS
1 Lor 23 Geylang Road, Singapore 388352. Tel: 7453969

Singapore Action Group of Elders (SAGE)
19 Toa Payoh West, Singapore 318876.
Tel: 3537159/1800-3538633

Domiciliary Care Services

Home Nursing Service, The Home Nursing Foundation (HQ).
26 Dunearn Road, Singapore 309423.
Tel: 2560078 Fax: 2561371

Home nursing centres are usually situated at polyclinics. Referrals to home nursing centres are made by the doctor to an appointment centre. Traditionally, the Home Nursing Service provides nurses who visit the patients at home for a variety of reasons: wound dressing, changing of feeding tube or urinary catheter, administration of injections, and so on. Recently, the Foundation started a home medical service where a nurse will attend to a medically stable, homebound patient at home, and then allow the family to obtain medication from the polyclinic on the patient's behalf.

Hua Mei Mobile Clinic
#02-01/03 Community Services Complex
Alexandra Hospital
378 Alexandra Road, Singapore 159964. Tel: 4716007

Touch Community Services
3615 Jalan Bukit Merah, 3rd floor Touch Community Theatre,
Singapore 159461. Tel: 3770122

CODE 4 Medical Services
Tel: 741744/7411144

HQ/East Zone
461 Sims Ave, Singapore 387541.

Central Zone
Kong Meng San Phor Kark See
88 Bright Hill Rd, Singapore 574117.

West Zone
The Singapore Buddhist Lodge
17 Kim Yam Rd, Singapore 239329.

Index